A Stroke of Help

A Stroke Recovery Journey

Alison and Phillip Bell

Thankful for God's Healing
Phillip Bell
Romans 8:28
2 Cor 1:4

ISBN: 978-1-63492-177-0

Published by BookLocker.com, Inc., St. Petersburg, Florida.

Printed on acid-free paper.

BookLocker.com, Inc.
2017

First Edition

Dedication

For the thousands of stroke survivors and their caregivers.

I pray my experience brings you encouragement and the strength to continue working hard and maintain a positive outlook as your recovery journey progresses!

In memory of Dr. Carl Schmidt, a heart surgeon and stroke survivor who was my HBOT diving partner for a few weeks. Dr. Carl provided me with the courage and inspiration to continue working to get stronger and better. I can only hope to possess a fraction of his courage, and keep his memory alive through my efforts to inspire other stroke survivors as he did for me.

Acknowledgements

First, I have to thank my Heavenly Father as He has brought me safely through the valley of the shadow of death, and blessed me with a great team of medical professionals. Next, I must thank my wife Alison as she has been by my side throughout this journey and has been the best caregiver I could ask for. In addition, our family Rachel, Chad, Jenny, Daniel and Laura Beth have provided me with an enormous amount of encouragement and the inspiration to not give up.

Finally, I do not know what we would have done without our neighbor, Mark Kramer, as he came to our rescue numerous times. Lastly, we have been overwhelmed by the concerns, visits and prayers of so many from our extended family, friends and church family that I would run out of space to start naming you all, but please know that Alison and I cannot say thank you enough for everything you have done and continue to do for us.

Table of Contents

Preface

We are at a time when the National Stroke Association, American Heart Association and many others have devoted countless financial resources and hours to increase stroke awareness and prevention. My experience acknowledges the importance of being proactive in taking care of your body in order to prevent high cholesterol, high blood pressure and being overweight, but sometimes all the education and awareness possible is not enough to prevent a stroke from happening. While taking you through my journey I plan to emphasize stroke recovery as there seems to be limited emphasis in this area beyond traditional speech, occupational and physical therapy by most of the medical community. My personal experience demonstrates there are medical breakthroughs that will benefit stroke survivors during their recovery journey that are either not being communicated or utilized, and I hope to help change that position.

The format I have chosen for this book is, for the most part, a chronological journal as I remember things unfolding rather than the format of a traditional book as I am far from an accomplished writer.

Due to being in and out of consciousness prior to arriving at Stallworth Rehabilitation Hospital I have relied heavily on Alison to help me share the most critical periods and events of this journey.

Introduction

My name is Phillip Bell and I grew up in the rural West Tennessee town of Milan. Milan is a blue-collar town located about an hour East of Memphis and two hours West of Nashville. I inherited from my Father a love for sports that will rival anyone. It is an everyday occurrence in my house to see the television flip from one sporting event to another. The only sports I do not follow are lacrosse, tennis, boxing, UFC, MMA and horse racing, except for the triple crown. My greatest enjoyment from sports comes from watching college football and St. Louis Cardinals baseball.

My Father was a self-employed carpenter, and once I was old enough to know what to do safely I started working for him. Being self-employed there were no vacations in the summer. Therefore, I grabbed my hammer and went to work too in order to earn my own spending money. When in college I worked every opportunity. That is, I was working during the summer and all the breaks, e.g. Christmas, Spring and any others.

I learned to work hard and to acknowledge the customer is always right. The customer always received a full day's worth of work and if anyone was going to be short-changed it was my Father. Another thing he taught me was if you do not have the time to do it right the first time you definitely don't have time to do it over.

That work ethic carried over to my professional career as an accountant.

Although I never gave it much thought my health was always good. My only struggle has been keeping my weight under control, but even that was nothing of significance. It continues to be a struggle today due to my lack of self-discipline to limit the calorie intake, and a physical disability that prevents me from exercising as I once did and enjoy.

Why I'm Writing

As someone who suffered and survived a brain hemorrhage and hemorrhagic stroke I have been encouraged by two verses of scripture, and have the desire to share them along with my story.

And we know that God causes everything to work together for the good for those who love God and are called according to His purpose. Romans 8:28 NLT

This verse from God's inspired Word is extremely special to me and I hope the words on the following pages will explain why.

He comforts us in all our troubles so that we can comfort others. When they are troubled, we will be able to give them the same comfort God has given us. 2 Corinthians 1:4 NLT

My interpretation of this verse is providing me with the reason God allowed me to survive the brain trauma. I believe I have the responsibility to share my story and try to bring encouragement to other stroke survivors and their caregivers. A former boss and member of my support network, Gary Wells, has encouraged me for several months to write this book in order to share my experience if I really do want to try to encourage others. Gary is one of the most optimistic people I know, and I am thankful he chose to share some of his optimism with me as his positive outlook is contagious. Although this project has been extremely painful as Alison and I relived a very difficult time we are hopeful it will provide comfort to others. Thus, here we go!

I have found there to be a high quality of life after suffering and surviving a stroke, but you and your caregiver have to take control of your healthcare and recovery. This could sometimes lead you to making decisions and taking actions your doctors might disagree with, but it is your life! I think as you read my story you will find several examples of where my wife and I took such actions.

Two Kinds of Strokes

According to the American Stroke Association approximately 795,000 strokes occur each year, and stroke is the number five cause of death in the United States, killing approximately 130,000 people each year.

There are two types of strokes, ischemic and hemorrhagic. An ischemic stroke is caused by a lack of blood and oxygen to the brain due to a blockage in an artery. This type is the most common type as it accounts for 83% of all strokes.

A hemorrhagic stroke is caused by a lack of blood and oxygen to the brain due to a ruptured artery, and is more commonly referred to as either an aneurysm or bleed. This type of stroke accounts for 17% of all strokes,[i] but 10% to 15% of those individuals will not survive. Another concern is of those who survive 20% will suffer permanent brain damage.[ii] Therefore, I must give thanks and praise God for where I am today! **Reflect on both verses of scripture.**

Although there are only two types of strokes, no two strokes are alike. Therefore the recovery journeys differ also. The type, side of your brain and location of the stroke will determine its severity and the outcome prognosis. In my case, as I said I suffered a hemorrhagic stroke with the ruptured artery being on the right side and near the brainstem. The brainstem is a very important part of the human anatomy as it is responsible for the regulation of the cardiac, respiratory and central nervous system, and is instrumental in maintaining consciousness and regulating the sleep cycle. Again, I must thank the Great Physician for being able to share my story!

Meet My Family

My story starts on July 22, 1979, one of the happiest days of my life as that is the day Alison Cantrell and I exchanged our marriage vows and started a new life together. As I write, thirty-seven years later, we have experienced many joyous occasions and a few that were not so joyous.

We both graduated from the University of Tennessee at Martin with degrees in Accounting. My professional career started immediately as an accountant for a manufacturing corporation in our hometown of Milan. The job market in and around Milan failed to support Alison's quest to find a job so we decided to start our family and she would begin a career as a stay at home mom. Our first child, Rachel, was born in 1983, and our second, Daniel, came along in 1987. Both of them have provided many lifetime memories, Rachel with her music and Daniel playing sports. Plus they both selected a wonderful spouse when Rachel married Chad, and Daniel married Jenny.

Rachel and Chad gave us our first granddaughter, Laura Bethany. **Reflect on Romans 8:28.**

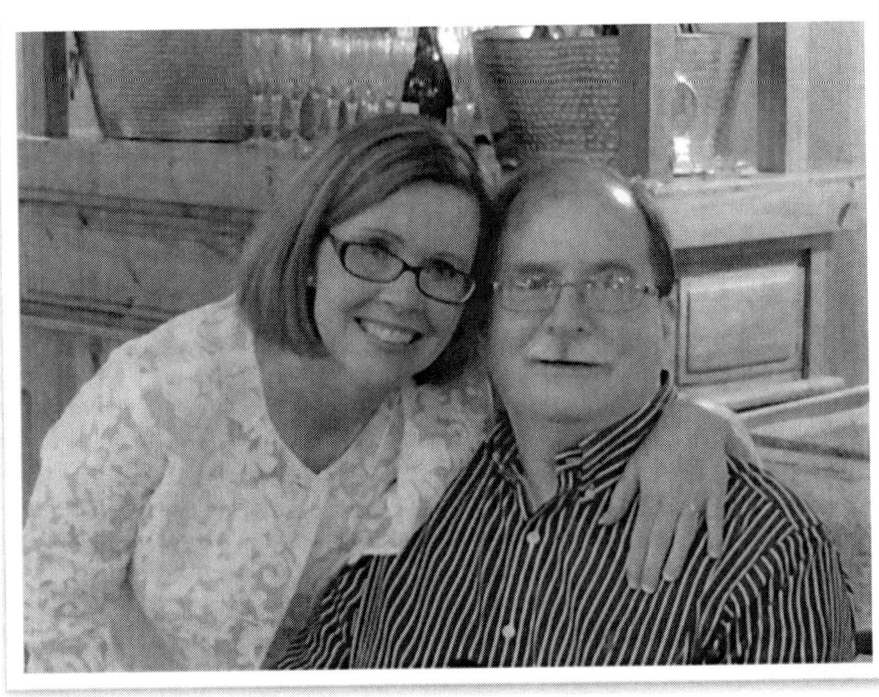

Alison and me 37 Years Later

My Pre-Stroke Work Life

My career as a manufacturing accountant was, in my opinion, very successful as I acquired my CPA license and progressed on a career path that I could never have imagined. My career has taken us from Tennessee to Illinois back to Tennessee then to Arkansas and finally back to Tennessee, all the while only working for two corporations even during all the relocation. In my last position with Black & Decker Corporation I was responsible for designing and implementing a standardized reporting package utilized by all of our manufacturing plants regardless of location. In addition, I was responsible for the review and testing of the internal control systems in place at our plants and distribution centers. While performing this role I also was tasked with identifying and correcting inefficiencies in our financial processes. Because we were a world-wide manufacturer with a corporate headquarters in Towson, Maryland, and I was based out of one of our Jackson, Tennessee manufacturing plants I found myself living out of a suitcase and traveling away from home 50% to 75% of the time. My travels took me to Towson for at least a week each month. Additionally, I was periodically traveling to our North American manufacturing plants and distribution centers for a week at a time. The most challenging trips were when I would go to Asia and Europe as those were a month long assignment. In Asia, we had a Far East Purchasing Office in Hong Kong, and two manufacturing plants in Suzhou, China which is about an hour West of Shanghai. The trips to Europe took me to a distribution center in Northampton, United Kingdom and manufacturing plants in Perugia, Italy and Usti, Czech Republic.

Unfortunately the recession of 2008 and 2009 had a negative impact on the company's financial performance that led to a corporate restructuring and elimination of my job. Thus a twenty-nine year career was temporarily put on hold while I searched for my next job. The cliche that hindsight is 20/20 could never be more true as what was a massive and devastating event could have possibly saved my life! **Reflect on Romans 8:28.**

My Pre-Stroke Wake-Up Call

Due to the constant traveling, eating out, and a sedentary life style my weight and physical condition had gotten out of control. One morning I stepped on the bathroom scales and learned I weighed more than ever before. In 2008 I turned fifty giving me a much needed wake-up call. I realized if I failed to change my lifestyle and take responsibility for my health I was at risk of following in the footsteps of many others in my ancestry and suffering a heart attack or stroke. As a result, this is what I did. I am confident medical professionals will say I got the sequence of events wrong, but this is how I implemented my self-designed program. First, I never smoked or used tobacco products giving me one less thing to deal with, and to get underway I started exercising. This first step served multiple purposes as it not only improved my heart health but also burned calories and served as a fantastic stress reliever. We already owned a NordicTrack cross country ski machine that I used sporadically, but was currently only collecting dust. The only thing needed was a good place for it to reside and lots of discipline on my part to get to work! I heard that if you can get in a new routine for two weeks you will make the new routine your new normal. I started setting the alarm clock for 3:30 a.m. when I would rise, go upstairs and workout for thirty minutes before starting my day. This became my seven day a week routine. When it came to eating, I did not go on a diet. I only stopped the in-between meal snacks and eliminated the fried foods, very difficult for a Southerner. I then started eating less red meat, but replaced it with baked or grilled fish and chicken. The final dietary change was to start drinking lots of water. These simple changes were not easy but they contributed to a forty pound weight loss! The final step, which should have been the first was to go to my primary care physician for a physical. My doctor advised that my blood pressure and cholesterol were excellent. He said I was in good health and should continue with my new routine. **Reflect on Romans 8:28.**

The Day My Life Changed Forever

A few months after losing my job we were home beginning to prepare for the Thanksgiving and Christmas holidays. It was Wednesday, November 25, 2009, the day before Thanksgiving and Alison was busy preparing for our family to gather at our house for a traditional Thanksgiving meal. Just before 2:30 p.m. I went upstairs to my office and shut the door because I had a telephone interview appointment with a prospective employer with a company near Memphis. I had a habit, whether at home or at work, of pacing the floor while talking on the telephone, and that is what I was doing that day. From my perspective the interview was going well, but then it happened. I heard a sizzling sound inside my head that was similar to the sound of bacon frying in a skillet. My initial thought was, wow that was weird, and then I asked myself what just happened? For a short period of time I still felt fine and continued my conversation and pacing, but then I started to feel lightheaded and nauseous. I sat down in my desk chair in hopes the sick feeling would quickly pass but it did not, and if anything it got worse. I continued with my telephone conversation and remember that I was beginning to slur my words while talking. I realized there was a serious problem when I heard something fall and hit the top of my desk. When I looked to see what happened I discovered my left hand, arm and cordless phone on the desktop! I quickly wrapped up the telephone conversation and called out for Alison to come help. Unfortunately, she could not hear me, but I was conscious enough to pick up my iPhone to call her. She tells me when she saw me it was obvious I had suffered a stroke. Luckily, Daniel was already home from college for Thanksgiving and he was rock solid, helping Alison to remain calm and staying with me while she made telephone calls to Rachel, our parents and friends. Initially, Alison was planning to take me to the emergency room herself, thus she called our next door neighbor for help. He told her time was of the essence and she needed to call 911 instead. Because I was slumped over in the chair and there was concern I might slide out the three of them got me out of the chair and placed me in the floor. It was at this point when I started to lose consciousness, but I remember them talking about whether they should give me an aspirin or not. Thankfully before a decision was made the ambulance arrived. Once the EMT's got upstairs they took my blood pressure expecting it to be sky high but it was in the normal range. They made arrangements to get me downstairs and into the ambulance for the short trip to the Jackson Madison County General Hospital. I remember hearing the siren, and then was unconscious until much later. During my period of unconsciousness Alison tells me we arrived at the hospital where my blood pressure was checked again. It was still in the normal range and arrangements were made for a CT scan of my head. That scan revealed the problem as it clearly showed a ruptured artery with blood spewing out. We have the CD of the scan somewhere in our house, but I never watched. I only know this from hearing the doctors talking with Alison several weeks later. This meant emergency brain surgery was needed immediately! A neurosurgeon was called in, and he set the stage for our future as Alison says his personal introduction was, "my name is Dr. Akin and I'm here to try to help your husband. I don't know if I can or not, but if I'm successful he will require months and months of therapy in order to recover." Fortunately during the introductions Alison was asked about my medications and if I had eaten. When she told them I had eaten breakfast, and I was on no medications, but I had taken a baby aspirin that morning bringing things to a screeching halt, Instead of going to the operating room for surgery I was moved to the Intensive Care Unit in order to allow more time for the aspirin, a blood thinner, to get out of my system. An intubation tube was inserted into my trachea while in the emergency room to help with my breathing, but as time passed I started to worsen and crash. Because my condition was deteriorating quickly Dr. Akin decided he could not delay surgery any longer. At eleven p.m. I was taken to the operating room for surgery, and two hours later Dr. Akin emerged as the surgery was over and I lived through it! Dr. Akin was successful as he was able to repair the ruptured artery, stop the bleeding and remove most of the blood accumulated on my brain, saving my life! After the surgery I regained consciousness, but was in and out due to the trauma and pain medication. Although the surgery was successful the lack of blood and oxygen to my brain caused me to suffer a hemorrhagic stroke. The stroke severely impacted me physically and cognitively. In essence it was as if my brain was telling me my left side no longer existed as I lost all feeling on the left side and was unable to walk or talk. In addition my vision was impacted as I lost peripheral vision to the left and was unable to focus my eyes consistently especially when the focal point shifted locations. In exchange I received double vision.

Alison Spreads the Word

A few days went by when Alison was home from the hospital for a few minutes. She, as she always does after returning home from being away, checked our telephone messages. As you would guess the inbox was full forcing her to listen to the messages. Included in the inbox was a message from the prospective employer I was talking to when the hemorrhage happened. He was calling to set up a second interview. I guess this means the telephone interview did go well, and he failed to pick up on the impaired speech I suffered. Alison called him back to advise I would be unable to schedule a second interview, and explained what happened.

Alison had to make a second call to another prospective employer located in Madison, Wisconsin. After completing six interviews and undergoing a psychological test I was a finalist for another job. Alison called the president of the company to let him know what had happened and that I would be unable to pursue their opportunity.

His reaction was more than you would expect as he expressed his concern and disappointment. Unexpectedly, his brother was an executive with a restaurant chain having restaurants all over the country. While I was a patient at Jackson Madison County General Hospital he arranged to have food delivered to the hospital from one of their local restaurants . There was plenty food delivered enough to feed my family and the nurses on my floor. Unfortunately I was unable to enjoy the food, but I was the benefactor of their generosity as I quickly became the nurses favorite patient.

Although I was at a different hospital this act of kindness was repeated on Christmas Eve!

The Neurological-Intensive Care

As I mentioned earlier 10% to 15% of those suffering a brain hemorrhage and hemorrhagic stroke will fail to survive. I made it through the surgery, and was moved to the neurological-intensive care unit. I was put on Propofol to induce a coma and prevent brain swelling. I was put on a ventilator during surgery to help me breathe. After ten days on the vent and because a ventilator is not a long term solution due to the probability of developing ventilator-associated pneumonia or VAP I had to undergo a tracheotomy to assist my breathing.

Once the doctors determined I had turned the corner to being able to leave ICU it was back to surgery to install a Percutaneous Endoscopic Gastrostomy (PEG) tube because I was unable to eat and the PEG tube would supply food and nourishment directly into my stomach.

The only thing I really remember from this time period is Alison, Daniel and our next door neighbor being with me during the ICU visiting period which was four times per day for thirty minutes each to offer encouragement and support. Mark, our neighbor, would always wet a wash cloth and place it on my forehead. It is hard to believe, but something that simple made me feel much better. My father-in-law would occasionally come in, take my left hand and ask me to squeeze, but I could not.

Alison and Daniel were well taken care of during this time by our many friends, family and church family who ensured they had everything they needed especially plenty food to eat. After the Thanksgiving weekend Daniel returned to college and Alison was on her own, but seldom alone as our friends and church family were always nearby. Unfortunately, Rachel was unable to be there too because she was in the hospital in Jonesboro, Arkansas fighting her own health crisis. Alison was really pulled as her husband and daughter were both in intensive care at the same time causing her to keep her cell phone in hand continually as she would receive updates on Rachel's condition from Chad and one of her doctors, who happens to be a personal friend of ours and a member of my support network.

Out of the Critical Period

After fully regaining consciousness I was moved to a private room, but I was very anxious and easily annoyed by sounds it was not only talking but things as simple as the clicking of an iPhone keypad leading Alison to limit visitors and causing my doctors to create a concoction composed of prescription medication that I received every night in order to help me relax and sleep.

Once the semester was over Daniel returned to Jackson to help his mom. He jumped on one opportunity to help. I have had a mustache since I was a senior in high school, and one day Alison decided it was past time for a shave. After finishing my face it was time to trim the mustache, but she lacked confidence to do it causing me to suggest she just shave it off! Daniel heard me say that and quickly said, "can I do it?" Nothing like a helpful son. Alison refused to do it and I still have the mustache today. She quickly developed the confidence and steady hand needed to keep it trimmed.

The old saying that "Laughter is the best Medicine" is true. For example, because I was still unable to talk effectively Daniel brought a small dry erase board for me to write messages. As I said earlier we always had friends lined up to make sure Alison and Daniel had dinner. One night a couple who we occasionally go out to eat with came to take them to dinner. The man, Johnny, came straight from work without changing clothes. When I saw him I asked for the board to write a message that said something like this, "Tell John R he looks like he's working, but he's at the wrong room," you see, Johnny's work attire is a suit and tie because he is a Funeral Director and I wasn't ready to leave with him yet! We all got a good laugh and recognized my recovery was starting!

Because I was unable to swallow effectively and still had the tracheotomy tube Alison and Daniel were taught how to suction excess saliva and secretions.

Once the time was right I was given a swallow test to determine if I could do so without the risk of choking and aspirating. I failed the test which meant I was dependent on the PEG tube for my nourishment.

A second swallow test was given later, but I failed to successfully pass it as well. Finally, on the third attempt I passed the swallow test which meant I could now start having liquids and small portions of purred foods by mouth.

Also after being moved from the Neurological-Intensive Care Unit and arriving in a private room I started to have some interaction with physical therapists. The extent of that interaction was extremely limited, consisting of the therapists moving me from the bed to a chair. While in the chair the therapists would exercise my arms *and* legs. They would ask me to do some of the exercises on my own, but I could not.

Because my trunk muscles were extremely weak I was unable to sit up in the chair for very long. In response to my being unable to sit up and being unable to do some of the exercises the doctor in charge of the therapy department determined I was unable and incapable of doing the therapy program required to help me. His reason was based on his observations and his assumption my insurance would not pay. Therefore, his recommendation to Alison was for her to make plans to transfer me to a skilled care facility. As usual Alison was ahead of her time because the May 4, 2016, issue of Science Daily includes an article in which the American Heart Association and the American Stroke Association strongly recommends that stroke patients be treated at an in-patient rehabilitation facility rather than a skilled nursing facility.[iii] Thus the doctor's recommendation was not well received and failed to sit well with Alison causing her to take the following steps. First, she told the doctor he did not know me like she did and he could not appreciate my dedication to work as hard as necessary and for as long as required. Second, Alison called my former boss at Black & Decker who happened to be the Chief Financial Officer. She told him that although I was still on COBRA she needed his help. After listening to her plea for help he contacted the Vice President of Human Resources and together they determined they could, should, and would help. They told Alison that Black & Decker would cover the cost of all the therapy needed! One hurdle cleared, and now it was back to the doctor. Unfortunately, or maybe fortunately depending on perspective, his professional opinion did not change, but Alison was able to acquire the attention and support of one of my nurses who agreed that with every passing day I was getting weaker and the recovery journey would be more difficult. The nurse was so upset by the doctor's decision that she was unable to come to work one day. The next day she talked with a social worker about our predicament. Together, with Alison's approval, they contacted Shepherds Center in Atlanta, Georgia who agreed to take me as a patient, but they did not have a bed available at that time. The second option was a HealthSouth facility in Nashville, Tennessee called the Stallworth Rehabilitation Hospital. Stallworth is very tightly affiliated with the Vanderbilt Medical Center and much more convenient for all of our family and friends, plus they allowed Alison to stay in the room with me while Shepherd's would have forced her to stay elsewhere. **Reflect on Romans 8:28**

Stallworth Experience

I arrived at Stallworth on December 23, and was welcomed by a Vanderbilt Neurologist, the doctor in charge of the therapy operations, and a team of therapists composed of a speech, occupational and physical therapist plus a case manager. This team was in charge of my care for the next eight weeks.

The team was not only responsible for my care, but they also made sure my recovery journey was started in the right direction and at the right pace. They were extremely aggressive in their approach as I was in a minimum of three hours of therapy five days per week. The weekends were reserved for rest, self workouts or make-up in the event you were unable to participate in a scheduled session. Shortly after my arrival at Stallworth I learned my neurosurgeon had prescribed and put me on an anti-depressant. He did so because his professional experience had proven that patients who had experienced major brain trauma or a life changing medical event transitioned to their new normal more effectively while taking the medication. My initial reaction was I don't need that, but quickly changed my mind as I was partially paralyzed and unable to talk clearly. Once I relented and accepted I decided I had two options going forward. I could either be bitter, negative and miserable causing those around me to be miserable too, thus avoiding me, or my other option was to be positive, smile and encouraging to others. The latter is the option I chose. Although it takes lots of effort and I might not always be successful, I do try, causing me to not always answer the "how are you" question honestly. **Reflect on 2 Corinthians 1:4.**

Once we were settled in after our arrival at Stallworth Alison received a valuable lecture from one of my nurses. The nurse observed Alison's tendency to try and do things for me rather than letting me struggle to find a way to do those things myself. The nurse sternly cautioned Alison that she needs to back-off as she might not always be around to help me. We learned several days later the nurse was speaking from a personal experience.

Also, soon after our arrival the tracheotomy tube was removed and the long process of the hole in my throat closing and healing was underway.

Speech Therapy: My therapist worked to strengthen my tongue and face by giving me tongue twisters to read aloud and sounds to make. In order to make these sounds I had to position my mouth and tongue such that they were gaining strength, She also attached electrodes to my face and used electrical stimulation to make the facial muscles stronger. I was surprised to learn that speech therapy was much more than talking. For example, I was given logic or reasoning problems to solve and in one session I had to take a stack of fake bills, write fake checks to pay them and update the checkbook. I also had math problems to work without a calculator and make change with play money. My biggest challenge was remembering the date and day of week, plus being able to read a paragraph without missing the words to the extreme left. Therefore, my therapist took me back to the time when I first learned to read emphasizing I use my finger to keep my eyes focused on the words and drawing vertical lines on the page in order for me to know when I reached the ends of a line. Learning to scan a line while reading was very difficult.

As I said Speech Therapy is a lot more than talking. My floor at Stallworth was devoted to neuro patients, i.e. we all had experienced some kind of brain trauma, and were a risk to choke while eating our meals. The Stallworth solution was called rehab dining where everyone came together and ate our meals while being supervised. Thankfully none of us ever choked but I continued this routine until the therapist decided I was no longer a risk. At that time I started eating my meals in my room. Although it was hospital food and definitely not as good as Alison's cooking, it was the best as I was no longer eating puréed food!

I determined early on that speech therapy had to be a priority because it is our primary means of communicating. I might not be able to walk or pick things up with my left hand, but I had to be able to talk clearly.

Occupational Therapy: This therapist worked to try to help me regain use of my left hand and arm utilizing numerous exercises to promote weight bearing and opening and closing my hand. During the entire time at Stallworth I was only able to open and close my hand when I was hooked up to electrical stimulation. If you know a stroke survivor you have probably noticed that most unconsciously form a fist with their impaired hand, and I do too. My therapist said that condition is called spasticity and I take muscle relaxers to decrease its severity. No luck with the hand and no luck moving the arm, but he did keep my shoulder from freezing up. He also made a hand splint for me to wear while sleeping. The purpose of the splint was to prevent my hand from forming the fist while asleep, preventing it from freezing in that position. Thankfully the splint did its job.

In all honesty occupational therapy was my least favorite and most despised therapy of them all, not because of the therapist, but because I was not experiencing the improvements I was seeking. Patience has never been one of my strong suits.

You too will probably encounter similar circumstances. It may not be occupational therapy, but one of the others. It is imperative that you continue to give it everything you have, including a positive attitude, and never giving up!

Physical Therapy: Before addressing my physical therapy I need to cover another condition the hemorrhagic stroke gave me. You may recall I wrote earlier my brain was telling me the left side of my body no longer existed. I learned at Stallworth this condition is common for stroke survivors and is known as left or right neglect depending on which side is impaired. In order to overcome this condition Alison was told she had to live on my left side forcing me to turn my head in that direction to see and talk to her. We went as far as to position the television so I was forced to turn my head if I wanted to see the picture! It took me several days, but I eventually learned that I would be greeted in the therapy gym with shouts of, "look to the left!" by the therapists if my head was turned to the right. Eventually I was able to overcome the left neglect condition, and face things head on.

My physical therapist was amazing as she was creative with the exercises we did. One day she too used electrical stimulation that allowed me to move my leg and bend it at the knee. Now, I learned long ago that electricity and water don't mix, so you can imagine my emotions as I watched my therapist put an abundant supply of water on the electrodes. She took me to the parallel bars with the electrical stimulation attached. That is when I took my first step after the stroke, a moment that was very emotional for Alison and me both! Recall my previous comment that the Shepherds Center did not have an opening, and that is how I ended up at Stallworth. HealthSouth has proprietary rights to a high tech treadmill for use by those unable to walk. The treadmill is called an AutoAmbulator. Day one with the AutoAmbulator was dedicated to programming the machine. Walking on the AutoAmbulator begins with putting on a harness that fits around the midsection and groin area. Because I was physically unable to put the harness on myself, I would lie on a mat while my physical and occupational therapist worked together to put it on me. Once done they moved me from the mat to a wheelchair, I then was rolled to the AutoAmbulator. With my feet positioned on the treadmill the harness was attached to a hoist. The hoist lifted me out of the wheelchair, and to a standing position. The therapists then attached robotic arms to my legs. These arms literally moved my legs when it was time to take a step. The treadmill was extremely sensitive to stumbles or missteps and would shutdown if encountered. Although the doctors in Jackson put my left foot in a boot to prevent foot drop I suffered the condition anyway. Therefore, my physical therapist fit me with an ankle foot orthotic, AFO, this particular orthotic was not custom made for me, but was an off the shelf generic type but it did aid in allowing me to lift my left foot when trying to take a step. With all of the setup completed and the logistics finalized I found myself on the AutoAmbulator daily, walking at a steady pace for twenty to thirty minutes. Finally, I was ready to graduate to another challenge. The new challenge was learning to walk with a hemi-walker. After I figured it out we would take extended walks to build strength, stamina and confidence. Some of my walks were limited to the therapy gym, but obstacles like cones, balls, chairs and other items were placed such that I had to figure out a way to maneuver around them. Additionally, my walking technique was critiqued and improved during my next therapy session. **Reflect on Romans 8:28.**

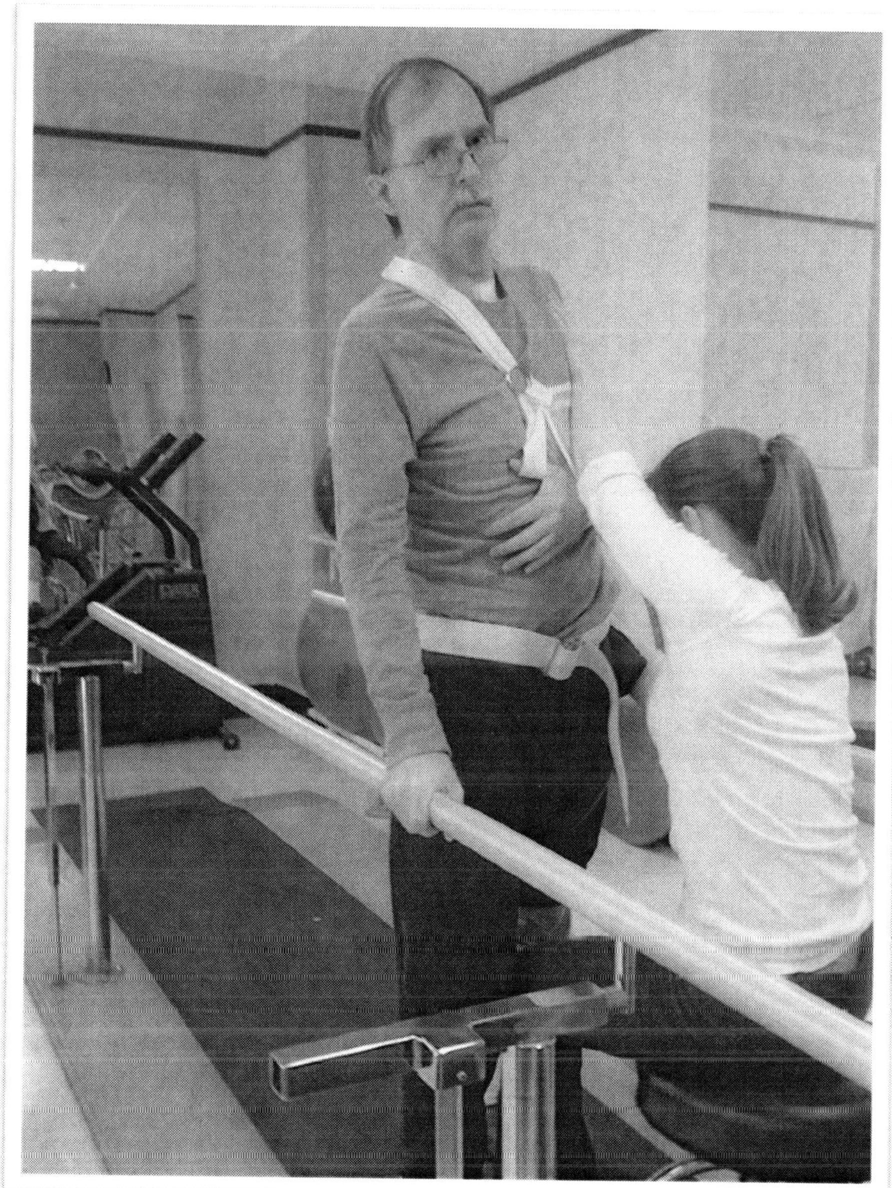

At the Parallel Bars Taking My First Step

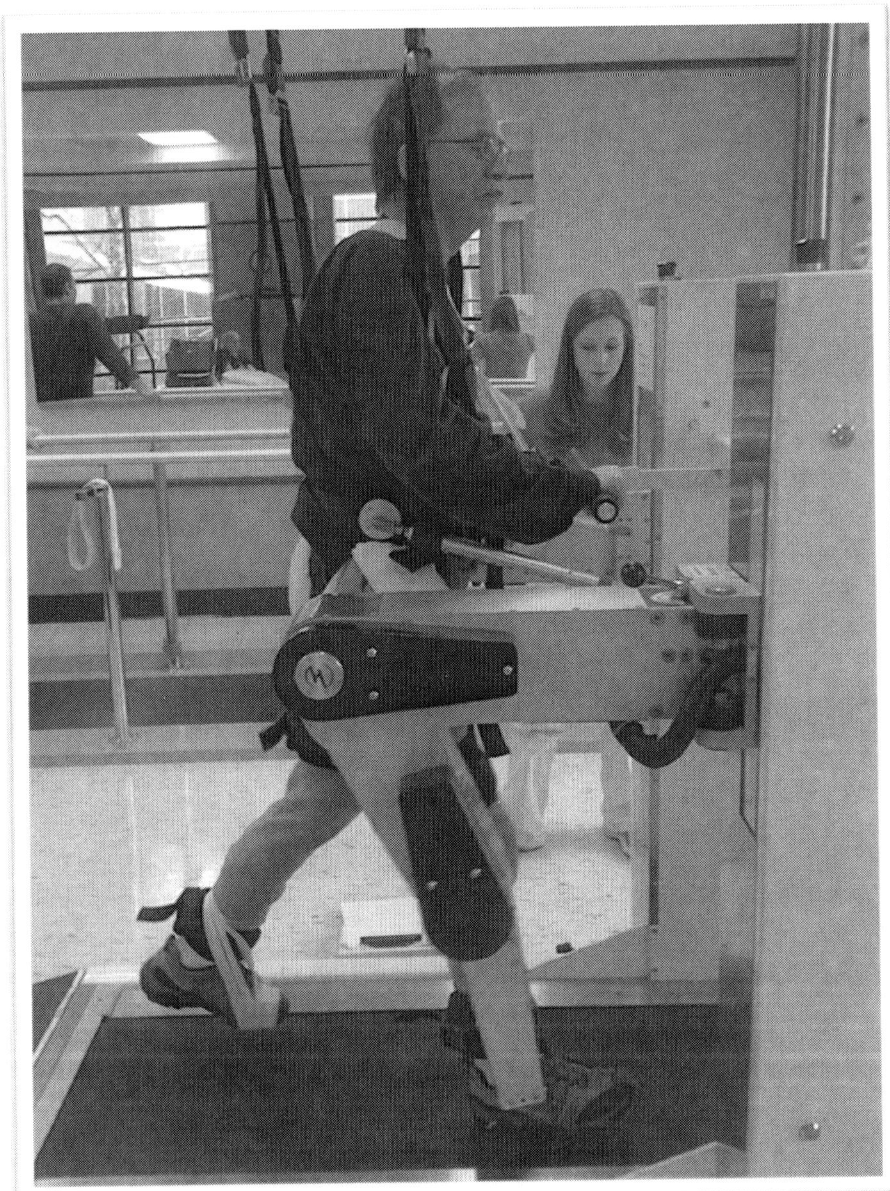

Learning to Walk on the AutoAmbulator

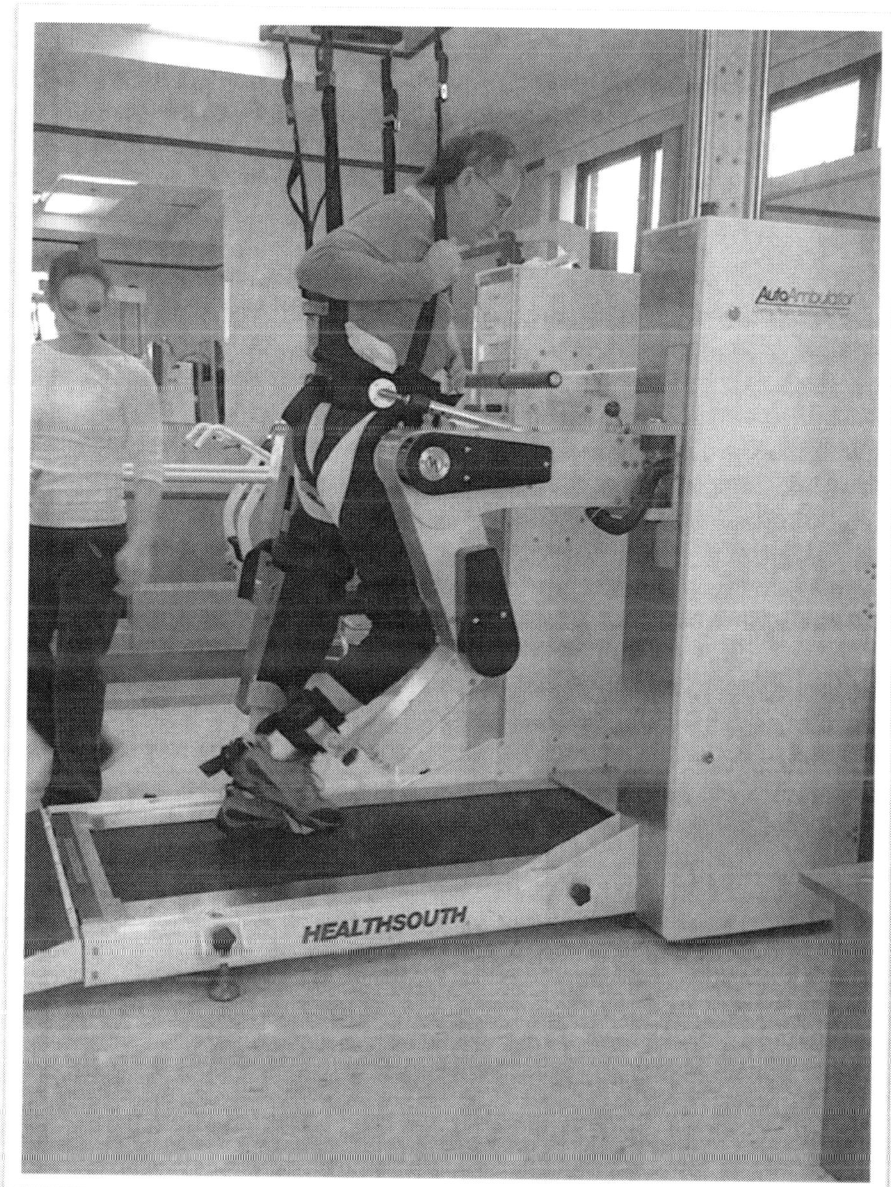
AutoAmbulator
HEALTHSOUTH

After learning to go up and down steps Alison and I were taught what to do if I was falling or in the floor and how to get up. It is called a controlled fall where she eases me to the floor without injuring either of us. Getting down was the easy part, but learning to get up and out of the floor was a totally different matter. We were taught how to get up without injuring Alison's back, and practiced this exercise several times.

Once all of their therapy program was complete we were asked if there was anything else we needed help with. We collectively said getting in and out of the car. Therefore, the next day Alison drove her Toyota Sequoia to the front door where we were taught how to get in and out. My therapist was thrilled when she learned Alison drove a SUV because it is much easier to get in and out of it than a regular car. The reason is because a SUV is much higher off the ground. Alison simply opens the passenger door, I back up to the seat and lean against it. Most SUV's have numerous grab bars to assist everyone while getting in and out. My next step is to grip the grab bar with my right hand, next I step up on the running board with my right foot. At this point I can lift myself up and into the Sequoia. The final step is Alison swinging my legs around and putting the left leg inside. She then buckles my seatbelt and closes the door. That all sounds complex, but after practicing with my therapist providing verbal instructions we got the process down, and now do it without thinking. Of course getting out of the SUV is much easier!

Sophia Comes to Visit

When I introduced my family I failed to mention our English Springer Spaniel, Sophia. We got Sophia to keep Alison company while I was traveling the world. Upon our arrival at Stallworth Alison was asked if we had any pets. When she told them about Sophia they recommended she come one day for a visit. All that was needed was to provide proof her vaccinations were up to date. Although she might not always demonstrate it, Sophia is a Canine Good Citizen graduate having done her training at PetSmart. Thus, Alison was confident Sophia would be on her best behavior if she came for a visit. Alison contacted the Veterinarian's office to request they fax her records to the hospital. Once her visit was approved, Rachel and Daniel made plans to bring her to Nashville for the day. It was a very eventful and emotional day for us all as it had been almost two months since she last saw me and vice versa. The first intriguing experience was the elevator ride. Once they reached my floor she hopped off and started down the hallway to my room as if she owned the place. Once she entered my room and saw me, it was an instant leap onto my hospital bed and then constant kisses as she licked my face from ear to ear. Sophia decided she had too much love to share so Alison took her for a walk to see other patients. At every door she would stop and look to see if there was someone in the room needing to be cheered up. Once our visit was done Rachel, Daniel and Sophia made the trip back to Jackson. That visit did us all a world of good!

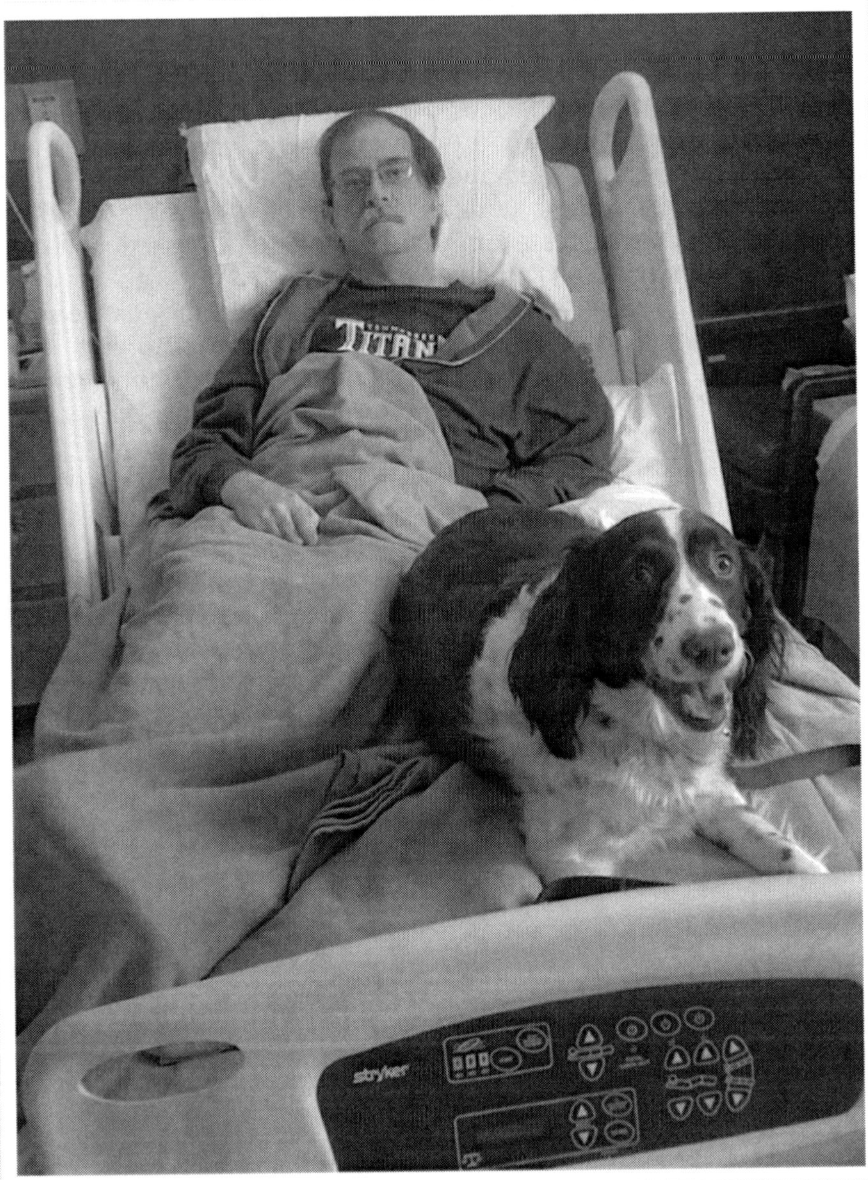

Sophia Takes Control of Stallworth

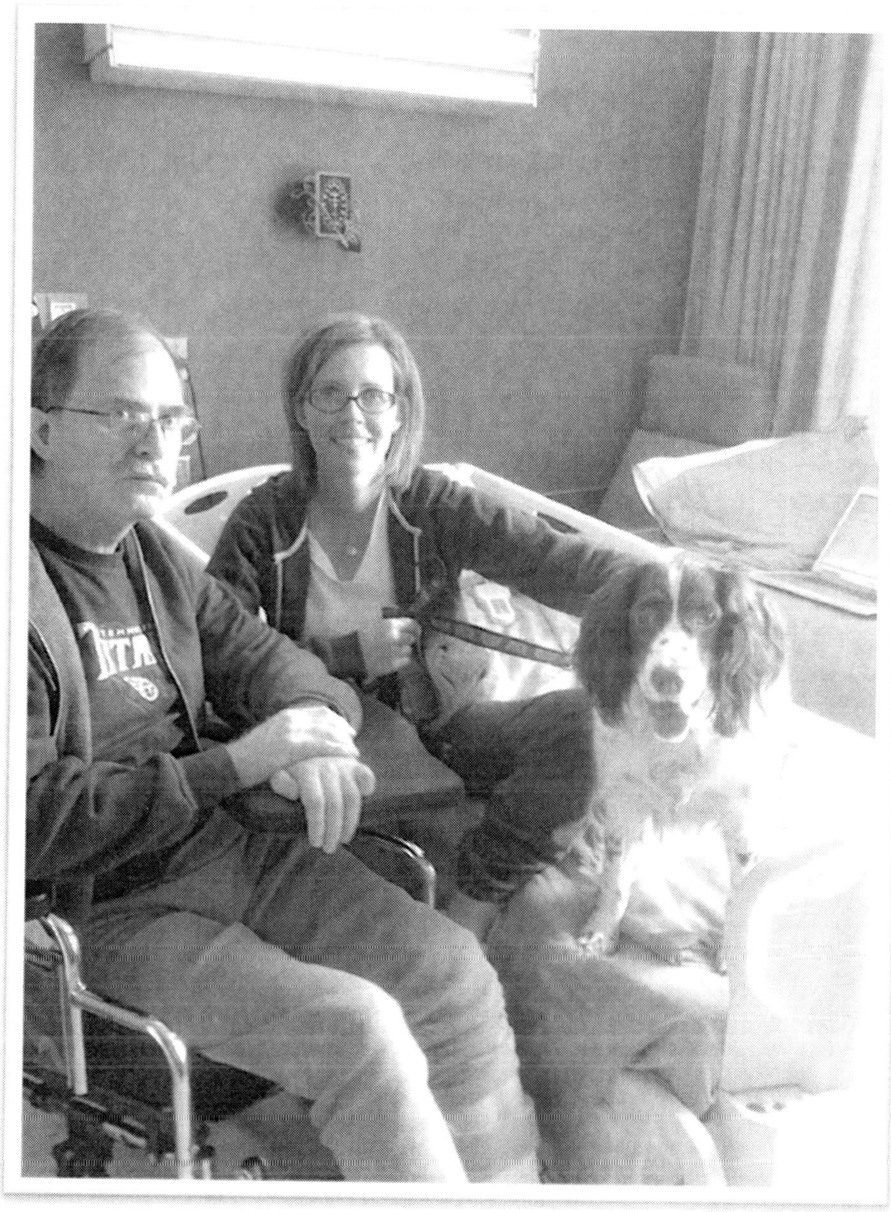

Let's Go Shopping

Before being discharged from Stallworth, patients had to demonstrate their ability to function in a public setting. One weekday some of the therapists loaded the patients ready to be discharged in a handicapped accessible van, and took us shopping at the Oprymills Outlet Mall. This was an overwhelming adventure because my assignment was to walk using the hemi-walker not only in the mall concourse but also in some of the stores. When I got tired it was acceptable to sit in the wheelchair allowing Alison to do the work of pushing me around. We also had a snack at the food court during a rest period. Once the rest period was done it was on to the greatest challenge of the day, going to the restroom! The therapists wanted us to find a handicapped accessible and family friendly restroom, and then take on the challenge of getting inside while sitting in the wheelchair. All I can say is, it was not easy and I am thankful it was not an emergency, Alison and I passed the challenge, but I'm certainly glad the adventure was not videoed. After that episode I was mentally and physically exhausted. Shortly thereafter it was time to return to our van and to Stallworth. Upon our return there was a debrief session during which we checked off the assignments completed and talked about our struggles.

That outing, although fun and not easy taught us we can overcome the unknown hurdles encountered in a public setting, but determination is needed, and we must pace ourselves.

Out-patient Therapy

After eight weeks of intense therapy the in-patient portion of my journey was complete. I was able to talk and walk with the hemi-walker, but I still had no feeling on the left side and could not move my left arm or use my left hand. In addition, I was mentally AWOL as I could read but did not comprehend or retain. The doctor in charge of the therapy operations removed my PEG tube as it had not been used since I left the hospital in Jackson. Although the procedure of removing the PEG tube was very painful and took my breath away, it provided a lighter moment when one of my nurses wanted to see my second belly button! My case manager helped Alison select a place where I would go for out-patient therapy. Together they selected another HealthSouth facility in Martin, Tennessee, called Cane Creek. Martin is about forty-five miles north of Jackson, and I went there three times per week for seven months. I had an hour of physical therapy and an hour of occupational therapy with each visit. During physical therapy I was able to transition from walking with the hemI-walker to walking with a straight cane. In occupational therapy my therapist was able to increase the range of motion with my left arm by taking her hands and arms to move mine, and we continued using electrical stimulation to open and close my left hand.

After seven months HealthSouth announced they were closing the out-patient therapy operations at that facility in order to focus on their in-patient services. This decision forced us to look for other options. We selected West Tennessee Healthcare's Sports Plus Aqua Therapy. My routine there was to continue with the three times per week program for an hour of physical therapy and an hour of occupational therapy. We alternated between working in the gym one day and then the pool the next time.

Reconnected

One day during my Occupational Therapy session Alison asked my therapist if she thought an iPad might enhance my recovery. I should have realized something was up, but I failed to put it all together. During my next OT session my therapist brought her iPad for me to check out. When I sat at her desk with the iPad before me I became frustrated as I was expecting my left hand to magically work if I could only put it on the keyboard. Not only did my fingers not work, I had trouble just getting my hand to the keyboard. My therapist recognized my frustration and suggested I use my right hand only. That suggestion led to more frustration as I thought I was giving up! Fortunately, I finally listened and used the right hand, that simple compromise opened the door because Alison, Rachel, Chad, Jenny and Daniel gave me an iPad for Christmas. Now I am able to send and receive emails, read articles on the Internet and read eBooks.

I share this story because making a compromise does not mean you have failed, but are just trying something different. Embrace a compromise, and explore the opportunities it presents!

Disabled

Shortly after my discharge from Stallworth and return home I had to face reality and accept that my accounting career was done. A twenty-nine year career was over as I was no longer able to travel the world or sit at a desk behind a computer for eight hours, much less my normal ten to twelve hours. Therefore, Alison started the cumbersome and time consuming task of completing the disability application with the Social Security Administration. Fortunately Alison's accounting degree came in handy and was put to good use as she was able to complete the application in a very timely and efficient manner that resulted in the approval of my application on the first submission. The next step was for me to request my CPA license be disabled also. **Reflect on Romans 8:28.**

Minor Setback Experienced

Due to all of the therapy I experienced a significant amount of fatigue resulting in my spending a great deal of time in bed. One night shortly after eating dinner I had fortunately gone to bed because without any warning whatsoever I began to seize. I have learned since that 10% to 22% of all stroke survivors can suffer a seizure for several years post stroke. In addition, a seizure is more likely to impact hemorrhagic stroke survivors than ischemic stroke survivors.[iv] Because none of my doctors warned of this possibility we were caught totally off guard and unprepared. I guess they thought the learning experience would firmly implant in our minds how to respond. Alison tells me the seizure became more violent and caused me to eventually lose consciousness. Once again our neighbor came to the rescue as he helped Alison turn me on my side and waited with her until an ambulance arrived to take me to the emergency room. While in the emergency room I regained consciousness and Alison explained what had happened, and that I was going to be okay. A grand mal seizure had taken its toll and it took a few days to recover. My Neurologist put me on anti seizure medication which I continue to take. This minor setback could have been a major setback had I not been in bed while suffering the seizure. **Reflect on Romans 8:28.**

Other Complications

I previously mentioned I experienced foot drop although my doctors had taken precautions to prevent it. My left foot was placed in a boot to keep it stretched and at a ninety degree angle, but that failed to prevent the condition. Wikipedia defines foot drop as a gait abnormality in which the dropping of the forefoot happens due to weakness, irritation or damage to the common fibular nerve including the sciatic nerve, or paralysis of the muscles in the anterior portion of the lower leg.[v]

As I said my physical therapist at Stallworth observed the condition and fit me with an ankle foot orthotic, AFO, but her AFO was a generic version and not custom made. Eventually, all of the physical therapy I was doing took its toll on this AFO and I was forced to get a new one. My physical therapist at Aqua Therapy insisted I get one that was custom made for my foot and ankle. The orthotist came to make the cast, and while doing so discovered my foot was not at the ninety degree angle. Therefore, an extra step was entered into the process. That step was to wear the new AFO without a hinge at the ankle until my foot was back to ninety degrees. Once the proper positioning of my foot was achieved I was ready for AFO number three. This new one allowed me to better lift my foot while walking. Unfortunately I now had another complication to contend with. The new problem was hyper extending my left knee while walking.

According to my physical therapist a hyperextended knee can cause serious damage to the anterior cruciate ligament (ACL) or posterior cruciate ligament (PCL) and cartilage injuries in the knee. As a result, my physical therapist recommended another trip to the orthotist. The solution this time was another custom made orthotic, but this one was more complex as it started on my thigh and went to my toes. This orthotic, orthotic number four, was a KFO and solved the hyperextended knee issue, but created another problem. Although the KFO did its job I was unable to keep the portion that fits under the foot in its proper position and in my shoe, thus the foot drop condition was not corrected. I even tried wearing high top shoes but that failed also.

Once again, my orthotist came to the rescue as he recommended I try a device called a Walk-Aide. When I went to the orthotist for a consultation appointment he put a demo model on me to see how it would work. I was immediately sold as I was able to walk without the bulky AFO or KFO, and I could do so properly, picking my foot up with ease! I was so excited that we ordered my own that day. The Walk-Aide solved everything but the hyperextended knee. To correct that condition I wear a knee brace in conjunction with the Walk-Aide.

The Walk-Aide is an amazing device to help those with foot drop. It is a battery powered device with electrodes . The orthotist programs the Walk-Aide to send an electrical impulse to my foot when it is time to take a step. The Walk-Aide is strategically positioned below my knee such that the electrodes can connect with the nerves in my lower leg. In essence it is as if my brain has been moved to be closer to my foot and sends the message to lift the foot when time to take a step!

My next complication is called shoulder subluxation which is a common occurrence after stroke and can be due to muscle weakness or spasticity. It is characterized by the upper arm bone, the humerus, dropping out of the shoulder socket. The muscles may be too weak to hold the arm bone securely into the shoulder socket or spasticity can cause subluxation by pulling the bone into an abnormal position. Both muscle weakness and spasticity can cause the shoulder blade or scapula to be abnormally positioned as well.

My occupational therapist while a patient at a HealthSouth Rehabilitation Hospital in Arkansas addressed this complication with creativity and success. In addition to exercises forcing me to put weight on my left arm he used electrical stimulation to pull the humerus into the socket. Once in place he used Kinesio Tape to ensure it did not slip out.

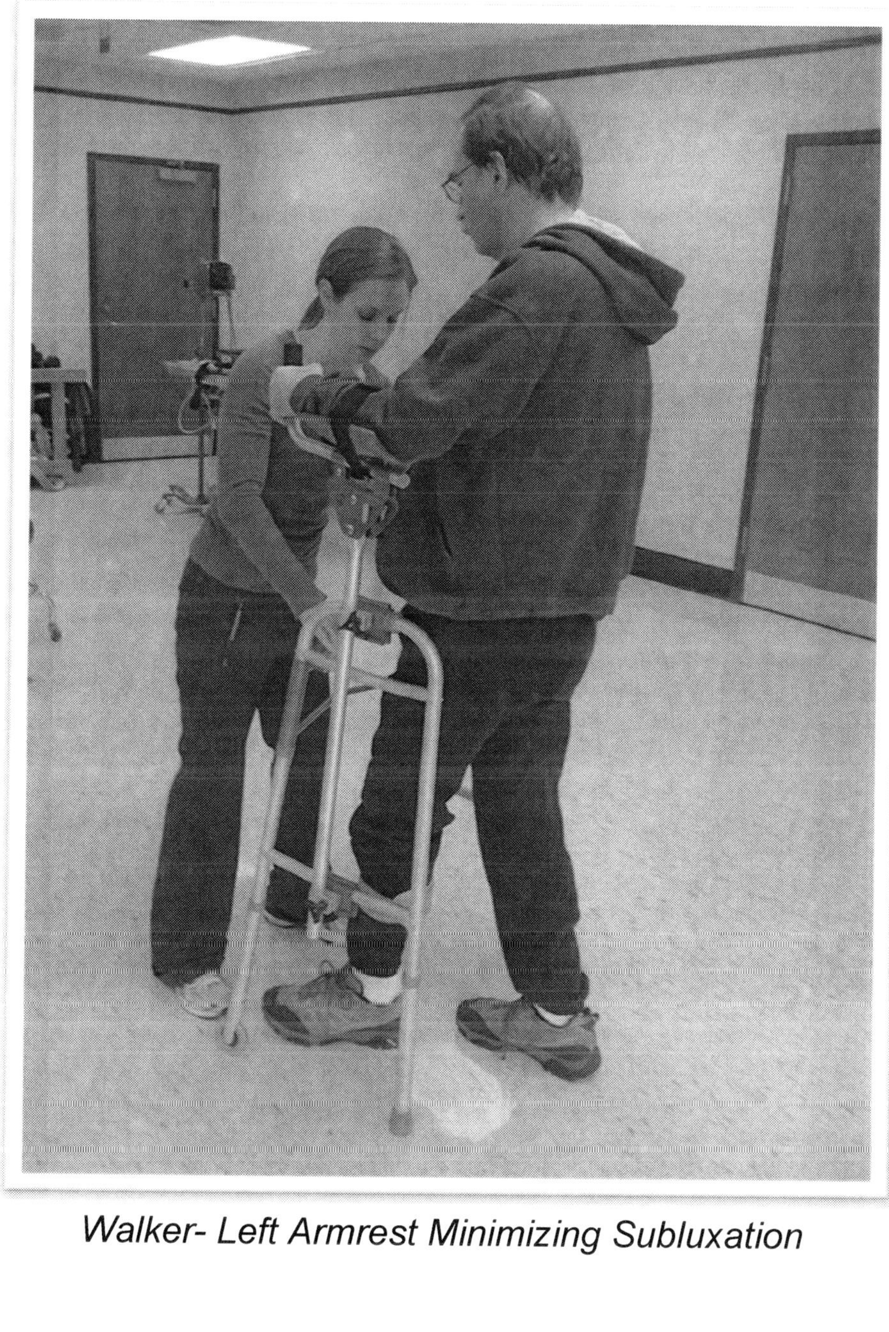

Walker- Left Armrest Minimizing Subluxation

Double Vision

As I mentioned earlier the brain hemorrhage and hemorrhagic stroke left me with double vision. This condition has not been corrected, but was made tolerable when my Optometrist put prisms in my glasses.

Although I have had several Optometrists tell me this is the correct course of action, some people asked, don't you need to see an Ophthalmologist for that condition. The question planted a seed of doubt, and I asked my primary care physician to make a referral.

When I saw the Ophthalmologist she recommended I see a surgeon from Memphis. The appointment with the surgeon was interesting for several reasons, but when the examination was completed he was honest enough to tell me he did not think surgery was the answer, and agreed with the solution my Optometrist had implemented.

Although tolerable I was still hopeful of eliminating the condition, thus during one of my quarterly check-ups with the Neurologist this complication was the topic of discussion. I was amazed and extremely discouraged when the doctor told us his solution. He simply said, "close one of your eyes!"

Hemorrhage Cause Discovered

My Neurologist was in search of what caused the brain hemorrhage. After ruling out completely high blood pressure he ordered an MRI with contrast. The contrast or dye allowed for a more detailed view of the arteries and veins in my brain. The detailed view led to the assumption I had a Cerebral Arteriovenous Malformation or Cerebral AVM. I call it an assumption because some of the evidence was destroyed during Dr. Akin's surgical procedures. According to my neurologists only 2% of all hemorrhagic strokes are caused by a Cerebral AVM, but both the Neurologist from Vanderbilt and my Jackson Neurologist were confident this was the cause. A Cerebral AVM is an abnormal connection of the arteries and veins in the brain. Normally, arteries and veins connect via capillaries, but in the case of an AVM the connection is direct. The condition is a birth defect which in my case was undetected. Once Alison and I heard the words "birth defect" our focus quickly shifted from me and to Rachel and Daniel. Our question to the Neurologist was what are the chances our children have this same birth defect. He assured us that the likelihood of them having a Cerebral AVM is highly unlikely, but the cost to run the tests in order to find out are very expensive and would probably not be approved by their insurance. I also obtained confirmation via Twitter from Walter J. Koroshetz,M.D. Director of the National Institute of Neurological Disorders and Stroke in Bethesda, Maryland. Over 50% of all Cerebral AVM's are undetected until the artery ruptures causing a hemorrhagic stroke. Those that are detected are discovered due to symptoms like seizures, severe headaches, or severe vision problems. As I said, my AVM went undetected and I never experienced any of the warning symptoms. Therefore, although my physical indicated I was in excellent health there was a hidden life-threatening condition waiting to literally explode! Now, I take you back to my earlier statement that losing my job might have saved my life. I say that because I could have been on a plane or alone in a hotel room somewhere on this Earth where English is not the first language, without help and gone undiscovered until it was much too late. In addition all the work done to improve my physical health made my heart and legs stronger while being forty pounds lighter improved my chances of walking again. All things really did work together! **Reflect on Romans 8:28.**

The Recovery Journey Breakthrough

We are now one year removed from the date of the hemorrhage and hemorrhagic stroke, and although I was talking and walking with a cane, I still had no feeling on the left side, unable to move my left arm, without peripheral vision to the left, unable to consistently focus my eyes, lacked energy, and was mentally AWOL. Upon my arrival for Aqua therapy one morning I was met by my physical therapist who was extremely excited as she wanted to know if I had considered doing Hyperbaric Oxygen Therapy, HBOT. We told her not only had I not considered it, but I had never heard of it. She recommended we look into it, and consider making a consultation appointment with Dr. Roy Schmidt, MD at the New Life Medical Group in Jackson as some stroke patients are experiencing benefits from doing HBOT. After therapy in the pool that day we went home, and Alison started her HBOT research. Her findings ranged from an instant cure to it is a farce and scam. However, in her reading she did discover a statement where someone said that one hundred years from now we will be asking; they, [the medical community], had the technology, why didn't they use it? That statement led us to make the appointment. During the appointment Dr. Schmidt was very detailed in his explanation of HBOT, how it works, and what might be accomplished. While I was at Stallworth I was told there is a twelve month window of opportunity to experience recovery following a stroke, and I was at that point in time. Therefore, I asked myself, is it wishful thinking that HBOT would help? Dr. Schmidt was very patient and honest as he made absolutely no promises, but said if I wanted to try it I should do a minimum of forty dives, HBOT terminology for a therapy session. He also told us HBOT is not FDA approved for stroke recovery and therefore considered "off label". This meant we were rolling the dice as it may or may not help. It also meant that the therapy is not covered by insurance or in my case Medicare. If it failed to work I wasted my time and threw my money away. Being accountants we are very conservative and cautious, and wanted time to make our decision. After a few days to think about it, I decided that although I would be Dr. Schmidt's first stroke patient, I was able to be his lab rat and hopefully bring encouragement to others. **Reflect on 2 Corinthians 1:4.**

How HBOT Works

I definitely cannot go into detail regarding how HBOT works, but my recollection from our meeting with Dr. Schmidt is that HBOT is a process where the patient breathes 100% medical Oxygen while under pressure. Ironically it was the lack of Oxygen to the brain that caused the stroke in the first place. The pressure is important because it forces the Oxygen to the injured cells. I was also surprised when Dr. Schmidt told me HBOT is one method of creating stem cells. Maybe that too speeds the healing and recovery HBOT provides.

HBOT Chambers

I have learned from my research there are different kinds of HBOT chambers, the most common is a mono chamber requiring you to lie on a bed-like surface that slides into a clear tube-like structure. This type will only hold one patient at a time, and you cannot fear being confined. The other chamber type is a multi chamber. The multi chamber is the type utilized by the New Life Medical Group. I describe it as a huge cast iron tank large enough to hold two school bus type benches and making it possible to hold six patients and a technician comfortably for a dive, obviously the way for those who have claustrophobia to go.

HBOT Dive Prep

Because you are in a high pressurized chamber breathing 100% medical Oxygen extra precautions are taken to avoid sparks. Although the chamber is equipped with a sprinkler system and the room has static free floor tiles, some of the precautions include: no makeup, jewelry or cellphones, but an iPad is permitted. You are to wear cotton clothing, clinic issued scrubs and no shoes. In a mono chamber the chamber itself is filled with the medical Oxygen, but in a multi-chamber it is filled with the regular air we have in any room of our house. The medical Oxygen is delivered via a hose system. Each patient wears a plastic hood. You have the appearance of an astronaut in training. Each dive lasts approximately ninety minutes as it takes fifteen minutes to pressurize the chamber, sixty minutes to breathe the 100% medical Oxygen and another fifteen minutes to depressurize.

As you will see shortly I have experienced numerous benefits from my HBOT dives, but you must recognize that doing HBOT requires commitment and discipline as it is important to do the dives daily. In order to receive the maximum benefit you cannot skip days or take time off until the series is complete. The only exception should be weekends. In my case, I started with a series of forty dives, and I was in the chamber forty consecutive days. My second series of dives again consisted of forty dives, but this time we went six consecutive days using Sunday as a day of recovery.

Your diet is also important as Dr. Schmidt stressed I should be eating lots of protein while doing HBOT. Finally it is important to stay hydrated, drinking lots of water once the dive is complete.

It is also important to recognize that HBOT does not replace physical therapy, but it supplements it and they are to be done concurrently. It was for that reason Dr. Schmidt referred me to Physical Therapy of Jackson in order for me to continue my out-patient physical therapy.

At this point I must pause and give special recognition to Dian Brown. She is a lady who I call the HBOT chamber wizard, working the controls to ensure every dive is at the correct pressure and the medical Oxygen is flowing properly. Plus, Dian takes a special interest in every patient as she enjoys watching her patients experience healing via Oxygen under pressure. When I first started doing HBOT I was physically unable to step into the chamber, Dian's solution was for me to sit in my wheelchair with Alison pushing me up to the chamber door. With Dian standing inside the chamber they would place my feet inside the door, and with Alison pushing from behind Dian would literally wrap her arms around me, lift me up and into the chamber!

My HBOT Experience

As you will recall before HBOT I had no feeling on the left side, was unable to move my left arm, had low level of energy that caused me to spend most of every day in bed, and I was mentally AWOL. After forty HBOT dives I regained the feeling on the left side from head to toe and regained limited movement of the left arm. Now, refer back to my comments regarding the Walk-Aide. Without regaining the feeling on my left side, the Walk-Aide would not have worked as I would have been unable to feel the electrical impulse telling my foot to lift up. In addition, my energy level was higher than it had been since suffering the brain hemorrhage and stroke. My time in the bed sleeping was over as I had enough energy to stay up all day, visit with family and friends and go out to eat! After experiencing these positive results I decided to do another forty dives. Unfortunately, this time physical improvements were not experienced, but I benefitted in more important ways, cognitively! I am now able to comprehend, retain and recall the information I read or hear on the television and participate in conversations. Another example is I am sharing my story with you now by putting my words on paper! **Reflect on both verses.**

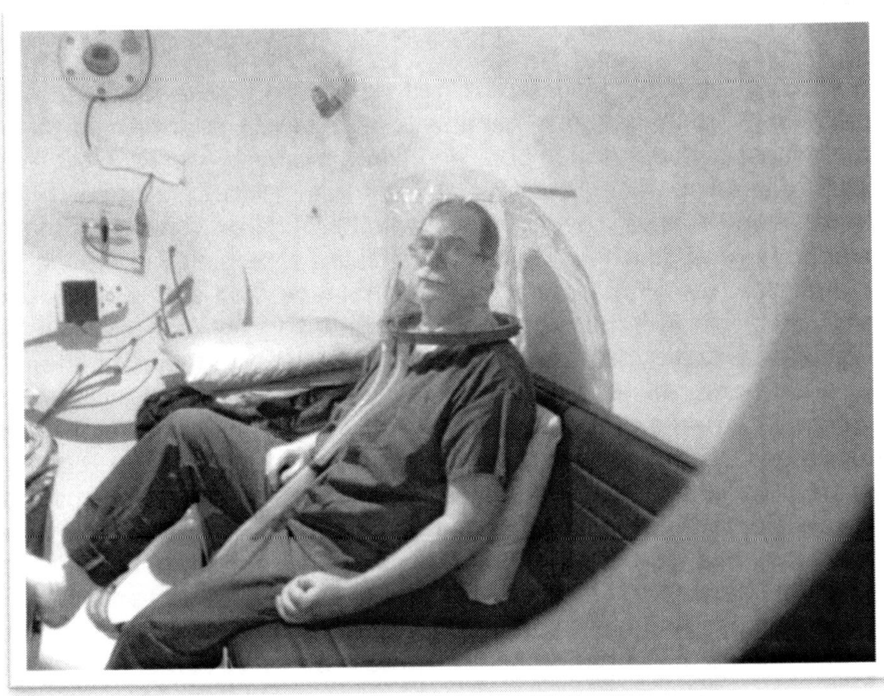

Hello from Inside the HBOT Chamber

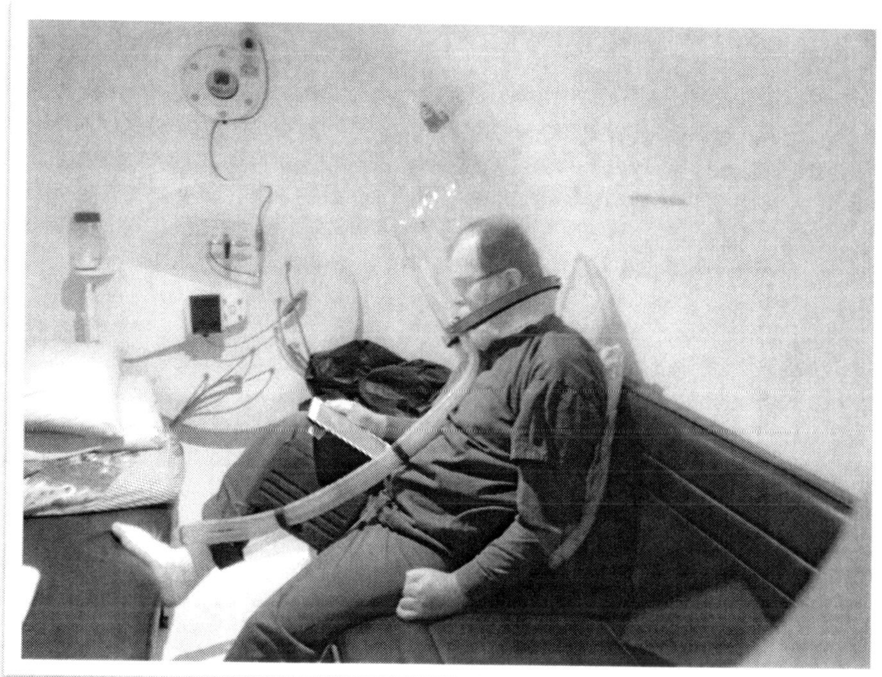

Reading a Book From My iPad During a Dive

Feeling Restoration Confirmation

As I said my feeling on the left side was restored after forty HBOT dives. This was discovered subtly when my left hand was itching after completing a dive, and being able to feel a comb move across my scalp while getting a haircut. The clincher was when I went for my flu shot. First, in 2010 when I went for my shot the nurse asked me if I had a preference as to which arm she give the injection. With little thought I said, "put it in the left as I have no feeling on that side!" She did as I instructed and we were ready to leave before I realized she had given me the shot. The next year after doing HBOT I had the subtle indicators the feeling was back, but when the nurse asked again if I had an arm preference. I wanted confirmation and quickly replied with, "put it in the left!" Well, she did, and there was no more doubt that the feeling was restored! Every year since when I go for my flu shot I always ask the nurse to put the injection in my left arm, serving as an annual reminder and celebration of the progress made during this recovery journey.

Doctor Reactions

After the eighty HBOT dives and during a regular checkup with my primary care physician I shared the cognitive and physical improvement experienced. My doctor was amazed by the change. After I told him I could not say the change was due to HBOT because I had continued with the physical and occupational therapy. His response was, "you might not, but I can. I have no doubt that because these improvements have been realized outside the twelve month window of opportunity HBOT is the reason why!"

My Neurologist from Vanderbilt referred me to a Neurologist in Jackson upon my discharge from Stallworth. Although I had quarterly appointments with the doctor I was not experiencing benefits. His examination consisted of me trying to push his hand with my left leg, squeezing his hand with my left hand and a few taps on my leg and arm with his plexor or as I call it a rubber hammer. As I said earlier I was without energy and mentally AWOL. This condition led to Alison doing all of the talking with the doctor as I was unable to do so. After the eighty HBOT dives and during a regular quarterly appointment I, for the first time, did the talking sharing my HBOT experience . Much to my surprise, the Neurologist failed to share my excitement or provide additional encouragement. Instead he stood up and walked toward the door, stopping only to turn and say, "You do realize there are no documented studies indicating HBOT will help stroke patients, don't you? I'm sorry you wasted your money!" I wish I had thought quickly enough to ask him, why do you need a documented study when you should be able to see the changes I've experienced, and aren't you excited to see one of your patients experience this kind of improvement? Needless to say, that was my last time for an appointment with him.

Since that day I have asked my primary care physician to recommend another Neurologist who might be more receptive to Hyperbaric Oxygen Therapy, but he was left speechless as he thought they were all from the same mold, but he did indicate there might be one on staff that I might consider.

Why The Reaction Extremes

I will never be able to explain the reaction extremes from my doctors with 100% accuracy, but I do have an opinion that could be offensive to my many friends in the medical profession, and will refrain from sharing. Instead, I'll list a few possible reasons that are purely speculative on my part, or were suggested in a recent Jackson Sun newspaper article, but I no longer have access to the article in order to give proper footnote credit.

The vast majority of medical doctors have been taught that brain damage is irreversible and is unforgiving.

HBOT is seldom taught in medical schools, but I do recall Arkansas State University hosting a symposium geared toward their physical therapy students where HBOT was on the agenda.

HBOT is used in hospitals to treat a number of other medical conditions such as wound care, but not stroke.

HBOT is not covered by insurance except for a few conditions.

For decades, HBOT has been discredited by celebrities making outrageous claims about its benefits, such as calling it the fountain of youth, but recently many professional athletes are turning to HBOT to speed healing and recovery from injuries, especially concussions.

Because Oxygen and the HBOT process can not be patented, there's no money to be made in marketing it.

Resistance to change within the medical community remains a major hurdle to overcome before the use of hyperbaric oxygen therapy becomes clinically available to the millions of people in this country who might possibly benefit from it.

A Very Hectic Day

Since 2009, November has been a very challenging month for me and my family, but that all changed in 2013. As I wrote while introducing my family Rachel and Chad gave us our first granddaughter. One afternoon in November Rachel went to the doctor for a regular pre-natal checkup, but learned her blood pressure was elevated, so much so that she was admitted into the hospital as a precaution. She talked to Alison that evening and we went to bed with the comfort of knowing she was in good care and being monitored continually.

The next morning I was awakened by Alison telling me to get up, we have to get ready to go to Jonesboro because we are going to be grandparents! After an hour or so to get a bath and eat some breakfast, Alison has packed our suitcase and started the chore of throwing our clothes, Sophia and me in the car for the two and a half hour trip to Jonesboro, Arkansas. I am convinced the four wheels of our car touched the highway twice that trip, when we left Jackson and when we arrived in Jonesboro! Thankfully the State Troopers were preoccupied that day and we arrived safely without a speeding ticket. We got to Rachel's room just as the Nurse Anesthetist was arriving to explain the anesthesia procedure for a C-section. A few minutes later Chad walks into the room carrying the most beautiful baby girl I had seen since I was in the delivery room when Rachel was born! Laura Beth had made her entry into this world. Both Laura Beth and Rachel came through the surgical procedure great! I was blessed to be there that day. **Reflect on Romans 8:28.**

I share this story because as a stroke survivor there are many joyous occasions you will want to experience and enjoy. You will need to work to regain your strength and reclaim your health in order to be at those events too!

Stem Cell Therapy

In 2014, Dr. Schmidt and the New Life Medical Group expanded their regenerative medicine offerings to include Stem Cell Therapy, with the stem cells created from your own Adipose tissue or belly fat.

Dr. Schmidt contacted me to see if I had interest in this type of therapy. As indicated earlier, I told Dr. Schmidt I am his lab rat, causing me to ask for more information. Alison and I made a consultation appointment in order to ask questions and learn more. Once again, Dr. Schmidt was extremely thorough in his description of the procedure, risks, and possible outcome. Again, the FDA is not onboard with this therapy so it, like HBOT, is non-approved and is considered "off label."

After taking some time to think and pray about the therapy, I decided to proceed with it, after all I have plenty belly fat to spare. Once I made the decision to proceed we had another major decision to make concerning the injection point. I had three injection point options to choose between. Either an artery in my arm, the carotid artery in my neck or the spinal column would serve as the point of entry.

Dr. Schmidt explained the risks associated with all three injection points. Being an accountant I am usually very cautious and conservative as I make decisions, but because of my relationship with Dr. Schmidt and because of his steady hand I decided to proceed with the carotid artery.

As an accountant we sometimes make investment decisions based on cost versus benefit, and the payback period required to recover the cost of an investment.

I looked at this from a risk versus reward perspective. Yes, the carotid artery carried many more risks, but the stem cells had a shorter distance to travel to my brain and their new residence so that was the option I selected.

On September 18, 2014, I underwent the stem cell procedure and immediately started a series of twenty HBOT dives. The injection into the carotid artery went smoothly although the belly fat extraction was a little uncomfortable. Once the injection was complete it was into the HBOT chamber for a ninety minute dive to ensure no air bubbles got into the carotid artery during the injection and to promote the growth, multiplication and establishment of the stem cells.

During the consultation Dr. Schmidt advised that it would take several weeks before I could notice any improvements. I continued to wait and anticipate physical improvements from the injection, and by October they started to materialize. As I listed earlier, some of the impairment I experienced due to the stroke was vision related. The stem cell injection allowed me to reclaim the ability to focus my eyes consistently even as the focal point shifted, and the injection restored my peripheral vision to the left!

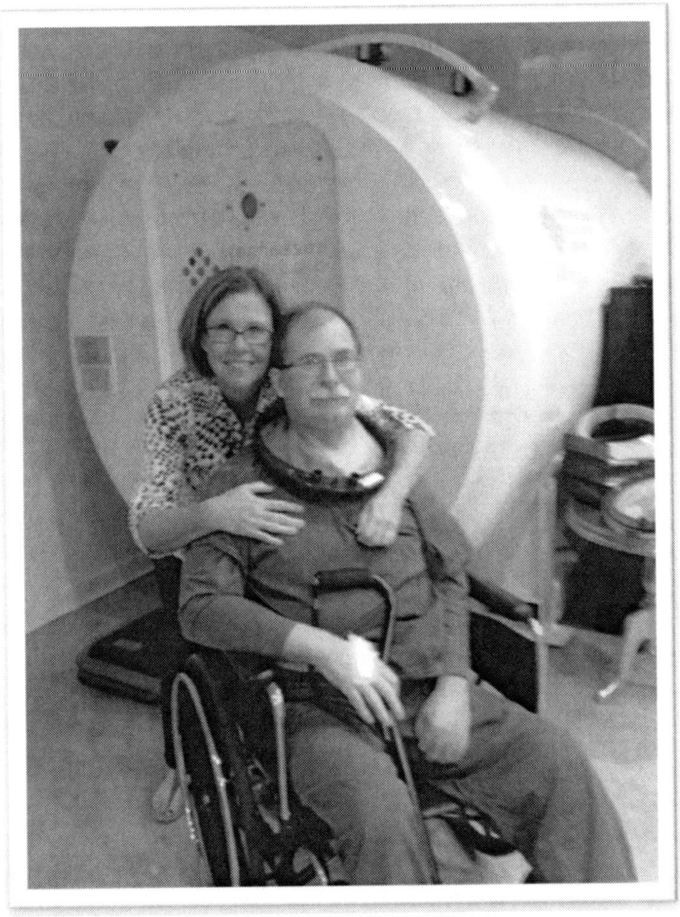

Immediately after the first Stem Cell Injection and Just Before the HBOT Dive

If Once Is Good, Twice Must Be Better

Due to the positive results of the stem cell injection I decided to do a second one. This time Dr. Schmidt insisted the injection point be in the spine. When I quizzed him as to why he cited studies from the United Kingdom that had success penetrating the Blood Brain Barrier, BBB.

Dr. Schmidt explained the Blood Brain Barrier is a filtering mechanism of the capillaries that carry blood to the brain and spinal cord tissue, blocking the passage of certain harmful substances.

I received the second injection on February 24, 2015, and followed it up with twenty more HBOT dives.

Again, after waiting several weeks I started to experience tingling sensations in my left leg, foot, arm and hand!

Can you guess what my Neurologist would think about the Stem Cell Therapy after his reaction to my doing HBOT? Unfortunately, he may never know.

At Home Therapy

Take a moment to reflect on my comment regarding the work ethic inherited from my Father. Physical Therapy, whether it is done on an in-patient or out-patient therapy basis is great and cannot be duplicated without purchasing the equipment and obtaining the knowledge and skills possessed by a professional and well trained therapist. However, it can be supplemented by working on your own at home. Due to the lack of a therapist to push you to exercise you and your caregiver will do well to develop the discipline to create your own at home therapy program. This program can never replace going to the therapy gym, but it can enhance. I have two things to share in this area. First, before I was discharged from Aqua Therapy Alison started getting in the pool with me and my physical therapist in order to learn some of the therapy program in order for us to continue after I was discharged. Secondly, we devised a program to be done in the convenience of our home. This program was simple and consisted of a sit to stand exercise. I did this exercise at the therapy gym but it was easy to duplicate at home. We simply took a straight chair and placed it in the middle of the room where I would not hit anything in the event I fell. I sit on the edge of the chair, then without using my right hand and arm to assist, stand up straight and tall after standing for a few seconds I slowly sit back down with a soft landing and no assistance from my right hand and arm. Next, at the gym I would do lunges either at the parallel bars or on a miniature trampoline. This exercise was designed to force me to shift my weight onto my left leg and foot while striking my heel first and rolling to my toes. To duplicate at home, we went to our bar. After moving the bar stools I would do the lunge exercise. Finally, my orthotist has two timed exercises he gave me in order to assess my ability to be independent and safe. We practice these exercises at home regularly.

It Started as a Joke

Jenny and Daniel set their wedding date for a Saturday afternoon during the month of April 2015. During my annual out-patient physical therapy in the Fall of 2014 Alison jokingly told my physical therapist, Joy Luy, that I had to get stronger as she was expecting me to dance with her at the wedding reception. That simple joke became a major motivator as the next thing I knew Joy had her iPhone playing music while she worked with us to dance! I definitely lacked confidence as Joy told me I was "stiff as a board" and was holding on for dear life. That was the beginning of what turned out to be part of my physical therapy program as we finished every therapy session with a dance. We, along with others in the therapy gym had lots of fun, but silently I was determined to make it happen! Alison and I started our search for music that was appropriate for the occasion and slow enough for me. After trying several songs we finally settled on Chicago's Just You and Me. When the day arrived I was not sure I could pull it off as I had been sitting in my wheelchair for most of the day, and I was lacking confidence in the left leg being able to support me. As the reception progressed our song was never played until Daniel's new mother-in-law, Patsy, reminded the DJ. That was all that was necessary as our song was the next one up. Chad pushed my wheelchair to the dance floor, I stood and Alison and I began to dance, or as some would say sway. The best part was Alison only had to keep me from falling two times. Regardless, it was a major hurdle cleared and a milestone reached as the tears started to stream down my face!

I encourage you to seek out your own hurdles using them as motivation to get stronger and improve your quality of life!

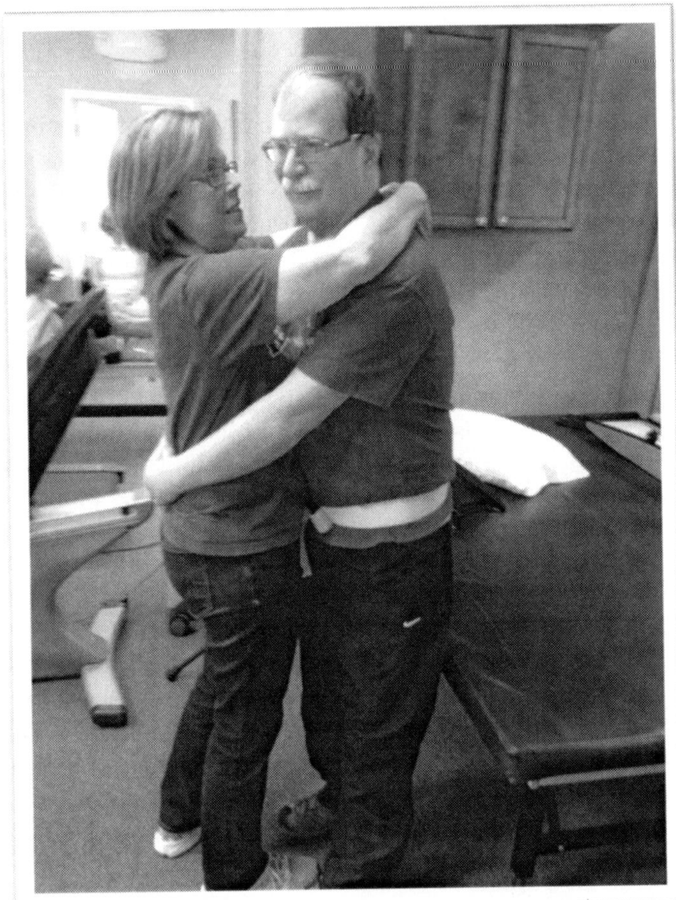

Learning to Dance after PT

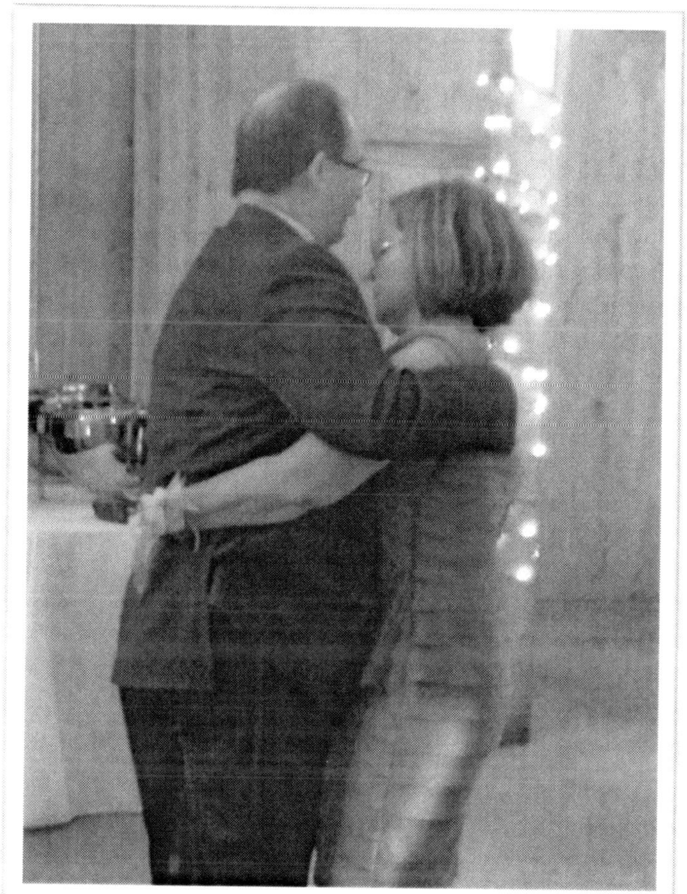

My Dance with Alison at Jenny and Daniel's Wedding Reception

The Challenge of Change

Throughout my accounting career I was always responsible for more than debits, credits and financial reporting. The most difficult part of my responsibilities was identifying and implementing change, otherwise known as change management. I quickly learned most people do not like change, and refuse to embrace it. It was my job to drive the implementation and acceptance of change. This required patience, perseverance and encouraging those resisting the change. Because I had this role I have been quick to accept change, until the hemorrhagic stroke. I now find it extremely hard to embrace change of any sort. For example whenever I got a new orthotic or started walking with the assistance of a new device, e.g. hemi-walker, quad cane, or straight cane. It would take me several days or even weeks to adapt and accept. The two biggest changes I had to overcome were new shoes and new glasses. It would have been much easier to throw in the towel and give up. Giving up are words not normally in my vocabulary so I was forced to practice what I had been preaching for many years.

This is just a word of caution as you will be tempted many times to cry "uncle!" Instead, you must draw from your source of strength, be that God, family or friends and continue on the uphill journey to recovery!

A Major Setback

In August 2015, while visiting our family in Arkansas I suffered a setback that almost closed the book on my recovery journey. After drinking several cups of coffee I started to seize. Alison found me in the recliner shaking violently. I remember her asking what was wrong, and replying with, "I think I need you". She immediately called 911, but for some inexplicable reason I stopped seizing and asked her to stop the ambulance before it arrived because I was okay. As you would expect, Alison did not listen to me because she knew something was definitely wrong. Fortunately, Alison was able to anticipate the seizing was not done, and soon after our brief exchange the seizing started again. The EMT's transferred me to the ambulance where I lost consciousness.

This was the beginning of a snowball effect that I could have never imagined. The hospital and emergency room were not far away and the seizure continued. While in the ER the doctors started an IV with some very powerful anti-seizure medication, but it had little impact! During that time I started having trouble breathing, and Alison was asked by the doctors about what they should do if my heart stopped! Alison knew my wishes because we both have Advance Healthcare Directives, and we are both Do Not Resuscitate (DNR). Although she knew this, answering the question was very difficult. She was finally able to answer as the doctors were getting ready to intubate due to the breathing troubles. Miraculously I started breathing and it was getting stronger!

Now, please allow me to offer a public service announcement, and that is to take the time to get your legal affairs in order. This includes a Power of Attorney, a Durable Power of Attorney, a Will, and an Advance Healthcare Directive as it is time well spent,. The Healthcare Directive is extremely important as it prevents your loved ones from having to guess about your wishes regarding the use of life support. None of us know when our time on Earth is done, only God does. By having the Advance Healthcare Directive you have successfully removed an enormous burden from your family.

Back to the emergency room where the doctors were certain I had suffered another stroke. This theory led them to order numerous tests to obtain conclusive results. All of the tests including a CT scan revealed that I not only did not suffer another stroke but all of the work Dr. Akin performed in 2009 to repair the ruptured artery was intact.

Two hours after the seizure started it was over, but during that time I aspirated . Also the ER staff ruined a perfectly good Polo shirt when they cut it off of me.

Although I was already on anti-seizure medication and Alison always made sure I took the proper dosage at the proper times the doctors increased the dosage and could not explain why the seizure happened in the first place. As I wrote previously, after the fact I have learned hemorrhagic stroke survivors are likely to suffer a seizure. This setback occurred almost six years after the hemorrhage, surgery and stroke.

Once I was transferred to a private room, the snowball I referenced earlier started to pick up steam. Aspirating on the coffee led to the development of pneumonia. My blood pressure and cholesterol had always been excellent, but for some unknown reason they were both elevated and I was prescribed medication to correct both. Next, I developed a blood clot in my impaired left leg causing the doctors to prescribe a blood thinner. Then, I started to experience acute renal failure and the retention of fluid. If that wasn't enough my ammonia levels were elevated.

All of these problems caused me to sleep day and night. Neither Alison nor the doctors could keep me awake which led to additional tweaks to my medication. Then, I started to hallucinate and talk foolishly. At one point I thought I had died, Alison told me I was very much alive, but I was convinced otherwise.

In my hallucinations we were starting a new fad with visitation taking place at the hospital rather than the funeral home, with everyone asked to wear the attire of their favorite sports team!

Finally, the doctors were able to get everything regulated, with my kidneys functioning properly and the ammonia level corrected.

My next step was to start physical therapy again as I had lost the confidence and ability to walk. After several days of therapy and walking with a quad cane I was ready for discharge in the opinion of one doctor who was much more concerned about statistics and the hospital getting paid than the quality of care I was receiving. Because we were two and a half hours from home my neurologist ordered I be transferred to a HealthSouth Rehabilitation Hospital for in-patient therapy.

The therapy at this HealthSouth hospital was identical to my Stallworth experience except for being updated with a few new techniques. While there I learned to talk without slurring my speech. I also learned to walk again using a hemi-walker. The one major exception is that I went through multiple evaluations by a Neuropsychologist. When the doctor came in to share the evaluation results and his professional analysis he said he was simply amazed by my cognitive abilities after the severity of the brain trauma I had experienced, i.e. hemorrhage, surgery, hemorrhagic stroke, concussion and two grand mal seizures. I shared with him my HBOT and stem cell therapy experiences, and he kept wanting to hear more. I finally provided Dr. Schmidt and The New Life Medical Group's contact information where he could learn more about the regenerative medicine taking place in Jackson, Tennessee.

One More Doctor's Reaction to HBOT

I must emphasize the negative reaction to HBOT and Stem Cell Therapy is not limited to Neurologists in Jackson, Tennessee. When I was in the hospital in Jonesboro, Arkansas my Neurologist started to walk out on me as I was sharing my HBOT and Stem Cell Therapy experience, but I continued talking and he eventually stopped to hear me finish my story, and even ask a question. Whether he truly listened or not is a different matter, but at least I tried!

Another Minor Setback

In November 2015, Rachel had to undergo surgery and we seized (not the best of words for me to use) the opportunity to go to Jonesboro in order for Alison to assist Chad with Laura Beth and taking care of Rachel once she was discharged from the hospital. One day, Alison left Rachel and me at home while she went to the grocery store. Although she was away I did what I always do when necessary, I got up to go to the bathroom, and for some unknown reason I became dizzy and fell. Fortunately my fall was backward rather than forward and I missed hitting furniture on my way down. Although I was without physical injuries I did suffer a lack of confidence as I walk. I had to get myself to a mental state where I was willing to "get back on the horse," and walk again. The next day I was able to overcome my fear and start walking.

You too may experience things that shake your confidence placing you in an uncomfortable arena. Be persistent and the sooner you try again the easier it will be to overcome your fears.

One Step Forward Two Steps Back

I title this section as I have due to continually making advances in the recovery journey only to be knocked off course due to another medical event. In July 2016, I suffered another seizure, grand mal seizure number three! Once again, although I was continuing to take my anti-seizure medication as prescribed the seizure broke through. This time I was home in Jackson, and the event required another chauffeured ride via ambulance to the ER and the Jackson Madison County General Hospital. Unfortunately, although I was home I was alone as Alison was busy at her family's farm picking blueberries. Whenever she had these outings she would periodically call to check on me to make sure I was alright. On this day I remember talking to her during a phone call and saying I was fine, but I did seem to be nauseous. That gave her pause and a reason to call again quicker than normal, when she called the second time I failed to answer and she returned home immediately. Upon her arrival she found me sitting in the recliner seizing. Another call to 911 was required. The ambulance and EMT's arrived quickly, but I was unconscious and partially regained consciousness as I was transferred to the gurney and loaded into the ambulance. I vaguely remember the EMT's talking to me, trying to get me to talk to them by asking questions. I answered some of the questions, but the topic must have been of no interest as I failed to fully engage. I recall arriving at the hospital only because of the jostling while being unloaded from the ambulance. At this point consciousness was lost again, but regained after entering the ER. The doctors were busy trying to stop the seizing, although not as violent as the one in 2015, the length of the event was almost as long. Alison tells me I seized for over an hour this time! The doctors started pumping me full of Ativan and it did its job. Once the seizing was done I had a CT scan of my head to check for any additional brain damage. Fortunately none was discovered. Once fully stable, the doctors increased my anti-seizure prescription dosage and I was later discharged to go home. It was either the after effects of the Ativan or the seizure itself that caused another setback. Due to my love for sports, especially college football, I'll use a football analogy to describe my feelings. The coaches have called a running play with the tailback, me, taking the ball and running around the right side of the offensive line just about when I hit full speed I am face-to-face with the biggest, baddest defensive end in all of football. He too picks up speed and squares his shoulders as he prepares to land a punishing hit and make the tackle. He hits me squarely in the chest just under the shoulder pads I'm lifted off my feet and driven backwards, slowly I have the sensation of being driven into the ground and thinking this is going to hurt, suddenly the back of my head violently makes contact with the turf! The contact is so that I remain conscious, but extremely confused and disoriented. The double vision is now much worse and I am extremely dizzy! The only comfort is found while sitting in the recliner or lying in bed! Because I'm not walking I am beginning to lose strength and confidence. With time, healing comes and the recovery journey begins again!

I share this story for several reasons. First, when I was discharged from the hospital after the brain hemorrhage, surgery and hemorrhagic stroke none of my doctors warned us of the risk for seizures. Now, I think I've written three times that stroke survivors have a higher risk of suffering a seizure, and I want you and your caregiver to be fully aware of that very real possibility. Secondly, do not try to do things alone, rely on God and turn to the medical professionals He uses to bring healing. I have learned some valuable lessons through this experience. Give your worries to God, and find a Neurologist who can provide the medical attention required. **Reflect on Romans 8:28.**

Oh No, Not More Complications

Since the last grand mal seizure I have struggled with extreme dizziness. I think this complication started due to the hemorrhagic stroke, but it moved to an all new level after the last two seizures. I talked to my primary care physician about the condition and he compiled a list of things to eliminate in an effort to determine the cause. The first item was to review all of my medications to see if there was one or a combination of the meds causing the dizziness. His conclusion was there were several of the medications that could cause dizziness, but it should not be to the level being experienced. Next, he requested a complete blood and urinalysis review. Again, nothing was out of line as the blood tests showed all levels within the normal range as was the case with the urinalysis. We then moved to my blood pressure which has always been excellent. Alison checked my blood pressure three times a day for a few weeks to see if there was the chance it had become elevated, once again, the blood pressure readings were excellent and revealed nothing wrong. My next step was to go to the West Tennessee Healthcare Dizziness and Balance clinic. This clinic contains physical therapists specializing in diagnosing and treating vertigo. An afternoon of tests confirmed vertigo was not the problem, taking me to the next step of going to my Optometrist for another eye examination. The exam revealed my prescription had changed so new glasses were ordered. When the glasses arrived I could definitely see better, but even after an extended adjustment period the dizziness continued. This took me back to asking my doctor to make a referral to a new Neurologist. When I saw this Neurologist I was extremely impressed as she had thoroughly reviewed my history and was up to speed on everything except my HBOT and stem cell therapy. Due to the latest seizure she determined it appropriate and safe to once again increase my anti-seizure medication and ordered an Electroencephalography, EEG. The EEG results indicated my brain activity was calm with no spikes which is excellent news, but it failed to provide any answers regarding the dizziness! As a last resort I decided to do twenty HBOT dives in hopes they might help eliminate the dizziness severity, but that failed also. Therefore, I am assuming this condition is something I will continue to live with, and it has forced me to park my straight cane and use the hemi-walker instead. I also use the wheelchair much more than before.

Although the stem cell therapy restored the ability for my eyes to focus consistently as the focal point changes, since the last seizure that has no longer been the case. I can still see the TV clearly, but reading is now a major undertaking again. This complication is so severe I am finding it more difficult to complete my writing, but I'll not give up!

Although not as devastating, it is my belief that a grand mal seizure is without question much more violent and almost as disabling as the hemorrhagic stroke!

A Word For Caregivers

Although you are not the one who has experienced the physical and mental disability due to a stroke, you have, without a doubt, experienced a life changing event too! There will be times that you will think I can't do this anymore due primarily to the emotional drain and physical demands that might be placed on you. You might also find yourself arguing with the one you are taking care of, or even be the recipient of what some might consider verbal abuse. I just ask you to remember that any verbal abuse directed your way is due to frustration by the one you care for.

While going through the many hours of physical and occupational therapy I have witnessed several instances where the therapist has received verbal abuse, causing me to gain an enormous amount of respect for all therapists and the work they do. Not only do they have my respect, but because they chose a career of helping people experience a medical recovery I decided to show my appreciation by working hard with them and without complaints. If I was tired, but the therapist wanted me to do more I would take a deep breath and push forward. After all, every therapist is only trying to help your recovery and make you stronger. I also found it helpful to have a sense of humor, kidding around when appropriate as it will help put a smile on not only your face and that of the therapist but also the faces of other patients.

If you are the caregiver for your spouse, I hope you will allow your love for one another and your faith in God to carry you through any difficulty.

In my personal case, I am blessed with a wonderful wife. Alison, on the very first day has been my very strongest source of support, motivation and encouragement, and she has never left me! Refer back to her reaction when the doctor recommended she make plans to move me to a nursing home. That spirit and love has never wavered. One of her requirements when considering Stallworth was could she stay in the room with me. She had the foresight to know she wanted and needed to learn how to take care of me! The nurses and therapists were all amazed as they had not seen that kind of love very often.

One day I was alone with my orthotist who had observed Alison for several months, leading him to tell me I was very fortunate and we make a good team. My response to him was I know, I am truly blessed and the words "in sickness and in health" are very easy to say, but not always easy to live!

I might be wrong, and I am confident Alison will correct me if I am, but I do not remember us ever arguing or saying anything to the other that we would regret, except for the time I had lost confidence in my ability to walk with the cane, and we were suppose to go out for dinner to celebrate Jenny's birthday. I had allowed my pride to get in the way and cause me to say I was staying home. Alison provided a much needed sermon that influenced me to the point of putting the pride behind me and walking with the hemi-walker instead! Even then, nothing was said that would cause regret by either of us.

A word of caution and I refer you back to the advice Alison received from one of my nurses at Stallworth, as a caregiver you will be tempted to be overly cautious and attempt to remove obstacles for the one you care for. For example, during a few of my physical therapy sessions my therapist would take me outside to walk. One day we were walking with Alison close by and she got in front of us to remove any rocks, etc in my pathway, but just as soon as she would kick a rock out of the way my therapist would kick it right back, leading him to tell her to stop as I had to learn to overcome obstacles on my own as she might not always be there to remove them. Yes, Alison can sometimes be just as stubborn or hard headed as me.

As a caregiver you have to also be ready to hear difficult questions that could be taken as insulting or offensive. For example, one morning I tried to see how high my head would bounce off our tile bathroom floor. Here is how it all developed. During a recent physical therapy session I was asked to sit on the edge of a mat and bend over to touch the floor, my toes or cones strategically located on the floor. During therapy I was able to do this with ease. Therefore, the morning I reference I decided in all my wisdom, to "help" by taking my shoes off. I was sitting in my wheelchair in our bathroom, and bent over to untie the shoestrings, only to find myself kissing the tiled floor face first! Once again our neighbor came to our rescue as he quickly came over to help Alison get me out of the floor. Soon afterwards blood started to come out my ears, causing Alison to take me to the emergency room again. The ER doctor determined I had suffered a "mild" concussion. Once things settled down and the emergency was behind us the doctor started asking me questions about my care. For example, he asked me in front of Alison, "are they good to you at home?" I quickly responded with "yes, very good!" I wasted an opportunity, but remind Alison of that event from time to time in a joking way. As a result whenever Alison accuses me of being hard-headed I am forced to agree with her assessment. It would have been easy for Alison to be offended by the doctor's question, but she recognized that it is probably normal protocol as they see all kinds of abuse in the ER.

Support Team

Although you have the support and encouragement from your caregiver you are on a journey to recovery that is uphill and on a very steep incline. Not only is the journey long and on a steep incline, you can see from my experience there are numerous hurdles to clear. For that reason I recommend you assemble a support network who will offer encouragement and pray for you too! After all, there is strength in numbers.

My support network not only includes my immediate family but also extended family, friends, former work colleagues, medical professionals and a wonderful church family. I try to keep them all updated regarding my journey by periodically sending an email letting them know what is happening. There are times I feel as though I am infringing on their time, but based on the feedback I receive in return most appreciate the updates.

It Takes Lots Of Work

As I mentioned previously a stroke survivor is on a long and difficult recovery journey. A journey that requires, as Dr. Akin told Alison "months and months of therapy" you must find an out-patient therapy provider who will work with you to make continual progress. As I mentioned earlier, Dr. Schmidt referred me to Physical Therapy of Jackson, and because my experience with them has been outstanding I use them to provide this annual service.

Medicare provides the disabled twelve out-patient physical therapy sessions in a calendar year and you should always take advantage and use them as an opportunity to get stronger and make additional improvements.

Everything Doesn't Work

Although I have been extremely fortunate throughout my recovery journey receiving benefits from just about everything prescribed or tried to help me. Unfortunately, not everything worked as I had hoped, and the same will probably be true for you too. I can think of two examples of where this happened. The first one was addressing the double vision, when I tried wearing a patch over my left eye. You will recall one of the Neurologists I was seeing suggested I close one of my eyes. I have no clue if he was serious or joking, but I failed to appreciate his suggestion. However, one day I thought what if I tried wearing a patch over one eye. Alison found an eye patch at Kroger and I gave it a try. I have to confess it helped some, but it caused more problems than solutions. The best thing it did was to help me look like a pirate. All I needed was a parrot sitting on my shoulder, and I was almost ready for Halloween. The second example occurred when my orthotist was working to become certified by a company called Saebo. Saebo manufacturers a device called a SaeboFlex designed to help stroke patients to exercise their impaired hand and hopefully regain use of that hand. My orthotist thought I would be an excellent candidate to help him become certified, and asked if I was interested in being his guinea pig . In exchange he would let me try the SaeboFlex for one month in hopes it would restore some use in my left hand. All I had to do was two hours of exercises every day where I would open and close my hand and also flex my left arm at the elbow as if I were doing curls with a dumbbell. I decided if I am a lab rat for Dr. Schmidt I could be a guinea pig for one month. Although I did the exercises faithfully it failed to restore any noticeable usage.

I share this because everything you try might not advance your recovery. The important thing is to stay positive, motivated and willing to try.

Quality of Life

Although I am unable to work, drive a car, go to sporting events, go on long walks with Alison as we would do while on vacation or shopping, or even get in the floor to play with my granddaughter I have discovered there to be what I consider a very high quality of life available for those who have suffered and survived a stroke. As you have seen from my story had Alison listened to the physical therapy doctor at the Jackson Madison County General Hospital I would either be in a nursing home or cemetery today. Instead, I have thoroughly enjoyed the additional time God has given me to be with my family as I have witnessed Jenny, Daniel and Chad graduate from Arkansas State University, the birth of our first grandchild, Laura Bethany, and Jenny and Daniel exchange their marriage vows where I had a dance with Alison during the reception! Thus, I say Romans 8:28 sums things up very well.

And we know that God causes everything to work together for the good for those who love God and are called according to His purpose. Romans 8:28 NLT

A Disturbing Trend

Now that I have shared my story I have one more thing to add. It may be my accounting background or the job I had identifying and eliminating waste in our financial processes, and therefore reducing costs, but my experience has caused me to observe a trend that is extremely disturbing, or at least it is to me. Our Federal Government and all politicians regardless of political party continue to voice their concern regarding the cost and quality of healthcare, but their actions say otherwise. Refer back to my foot drop complication as an example. I was fit with four orthotics that were covered by insurance and Medicare. Although these orthotics were covered, they all failed to work successfully. Ironically, the Walk-Aide solution that was successful is not covered by insurance or Medicare because it is not approved by the Food and Drug Administration. In addition, my Hyperbaric Oxygen Therapy and Stem Cell Therapy solutions have had the greatest and most effective impact on my recovery journey, but neither are covered by insurance or Medicare because they are not FDA approved either. The lack of coverage translates to many being unable to obtain this type of care or experience the same quality of healthcare I have experienced. Apparently, the FDA would rather have doctors prescribing medication and devices that do not work than helping people in need. It is for that reason I check all the legislation introduced in Congress in DC, and write my Representative and Senators where HBOT or Stem Cell Therapy is applicable. (No extra charge for my very opinionated perspective!)

The Next Chapter

Where do I go from here? If you recall one of my reasons for writing comes from **2 Corinthians 1:4** as I believe I have a responsibility to try to bring encouragement to other stroke survivors and their caregivers. How is this to be done you might ask. In all honesty I'm not sure but if you read and believe this verse:

You can make many plans, but the LORD's purpose will prevail. Proverbs 19:21 NLT

God will show me the way! Before closing I need to eliminate any possible confusion I might have created.

If my story has caused you to conclude I am anti-doctor or medical profession then I have failed. I have the greatest respect for the men and women who chose to help others by selecting a career in the medical profession. Whether a Neurosurgeon, primary care physician, HBOT chamber wizard, speech therapist, physical therapist or nurse, together they form a medical team that God uses to take care of us! However, I do have the belief that if you are not advancing in your recovery journey it might be time for you to call timeout and research other options, be it a different doctor, therapy gym or a controversial medical breakthrough.

As I am confident you have discovered I am a very active and passionate promoter of Hyperbaric Oxygen Therapy. So much so that as I write I have completed two hundred nineteen dives at the New Life Medical Group in Jackson, Tennessee. The first eighty dives made the greatest contribution to my recovery, as did the twenty dives completed with each stem cell injection. All the other dives I classify as maintenance dives. Just as I indicated earlier, you should do out-patient physical therapy annually in order to get stronger. I treat myself with an early Christmas gift of twenty HBOT dives each October as I have discovered they provide a boost of energy and make me stronger so I can enjoy Thanksgiving and Christmas with my family. I encourage you to also take control of your recovery journey and start living your life again!

Although HBOT and Stem Cell Therapy were right for me, delivering recovery advancements I never dreamed possible when I started. I have talked with many stroke survivors about my HBOT and Stem Cell Therapy, and without exception they always ask,"do you think HBOT will help me too?" To which my only response is, I can only share what they did for me and not what they will do for you. As I wrote earlier no two strokes are alike nor are the recovery journeys. I can only share what they did for me, and encourage you to give them serious consideration if you are unsatisfied with the recovery progress you have made or want to go farther than where traditional speech, occupational and physical therapy alone have taken you.

Notes

[i] Impact of Stroke (Stroke Statistics), strokeassociation.org, June 6,2016.
[ii] What is an Arteriovenous Malformation (AVM)?, strokeassociation.org, June 20,2014.
[iii] In-patient rehab recommended over nursing homes for stroke rehab, sciencedaily.com, May 4, 2016.
[iv] Walt Kilcullen, Seizures After a Stroke, strokenetwork.org, January 2014.
[v] Foot Drop, Wikipedia.org, March 23,2013.

CPSIA information can be obtained
at www.ICGtesting.com
Printed in the USA
LVOW11s1007210317
527929LV00001B/27/P